MENTAL AND PHYSICAL HANDICAPS IN CONNECTION

WITH OVERRIPENESS OVOPATHY

Mental and Physical Handicaps in connection with Overripeness Ovopathy

P. H. JONGBLOET M. D.

1971

H. E. STENFERT KROESE N.V. — LEIDEN

ISBN-13: 978-90-207-0315-3   e-ISBN-13: 978-94-010-2958-2
DOI: 10.1007/978-94-010-2958-2

TABLE OF CONTENTS

ERRATA

pg.   2, lines 25 and 26: *an aselect* sample read *a random* sample.

pg. 26, line 34: *an aselect population group* read *a random sample.*

pg. 69,   : Table 4: total no. per month in Oct.: *55* read *5.*

pg. 83, line 30: *not* has to be comitted.

pg. 103, line 5: Table *II* read Table *I.*

pg. 118, line 11: *an aselect population group* read *a random sample.*

pg. 122, line 11: Table *1* read Table *2.*

pg. 132, line 11: monoamino read monoamine.

INTRODUCTION

Parents of children born with mental or physical handicaps, tend to face the physician with questions about the origin of the abnormality concerned and the chance of having another child with the same condition. The physician then finds himself in a difficult situation since the causes of the majority of congenital abnormalities remain as yet unknown. In most cases he has to restrict himself to a mere enumeration of the signs and symptoms encountered or, at best, to a classification of the syndrome at hand. Efforts are frequently made to connect both the somatic aberrations and the mental deficiency with complications during the later stages of pregnancy, at the time of delivery or in the immediate postnatal period. However, a careful search for such items as abnormal dermatoglyphs, or 'degenerative stigmata', and, in particular, a post-mortem examination of the brain, often indicates that the handicap concerned should be ascribed to factors operating long before the time of birth.

Theoretically, the causes of abnormalities present at birth can be listed as of a genetic, germinal or peristatic nature. During the past decades special attention has been paid to both genetic and peristatic factors. The purpose of this thesis is to stress the importance of germinal factors, in particular those which, at least in theory, might lead to disturbances in the ripening process of the human egg. We were put on this track by some data concerning the circumstances under which one of our patients presumably had been conceived.

In March 1967, namely, we were confronted with a child presenting the classical symptoms of Goldenhar's syndrome, one of the syndromes showing a high degree of variability and for which a genetic origin is, according to the literature, unlikely. Therefore it seemed logical to search for exogenous causal factors operating during the early stages of the formation of the embryo. It was learnt that the child had been conceived in spite of application of the calendar rhythmic method; to be exact, towards the end of the second so-called 'safe period' of the menstrual cycle. The cycle concerned happened to be the first one after birth of the preceding child, a situation in which menstrual irregularities are not uncommon and in which ovulation may be overdue. Moreover, another pregnancy, occurring while the couple still practised rigid periodic abstinence, had terminated in spontaneous abortion.

Now experiments with amphibian and mammalian eggs, allowed to become overripe before fertilization, frequently result in either a nonviable conceptus or a malformed one (a.o. PFLÜGER 1882, WITSCHI 1952, MIKAMO 1968). This led us to formulate the following questions:

1. Does there exist in Man too, a connection between fertilization of an overripe egg and abnormal development of the embryo?

2. Are there fluent transitions in degree of severity of developmental anomalies, the result being spontaneous abortion, or stillbirth, or a live-born child with congenital malformations?

Though there are still many gaps in our knowledge of the physiology and pathophysiology of human reproduction, the above-mentioned animal experiments seemed to us to provide a suitable basis to approach these problems. Obviously, data derived from experiments with certain animal species cannot simply be applied to other species, and certainly not to Man, but they may lead to the formulation of fruitful working hypotheses. Accordingly, we began our studies on the assumption that the above questions could be answered in the affirmative (Chapter I). Perusal of the literature did not bring to light convincing evidence that this assumption was either false or true. Therefore we started our investigations by questioning 127 couples with one or more mentally retarded children, many of whom had connatal physical handicaps also. The interrogation concerned the time of and the circumstances under which both their normal and their deficient children had been conceived (Chapter II). This was followed up by a similar enquiry conducted in an a-select sample of 155 couples from two towns in the neighbourhood (Chapter III). In all groups where, on theoretical grounds, overripeness of the egg might be expected ('high-risk conception groups'), an increased percentage of spontaneous abortions, still-births and children with developmental abnormalities was established. These findings therefore lent support to our hypotheses. Admittedly, conclusions derived from retrospective enquiries into possible failures of the application of the calendar rhythmic method possess the inherent weakness of being subject to faulty human memory. In other 'high-risk conception groups', however, such as those with either a very short, or an unintendedly long interval between conceptions, such weakness hardly plays a role. Obviously, these our findings are in need of further confirmation. They do not offer irrefutable proof that overripeness of the egg may lead to developmental anomalies in the human being also. They may, however, be considered to adduce circumstantial evidence, which, combined with observations culled from the pertinent literature, justify the concept of overripeness ovopathy as a working hypothesis.

This concept motivated us to present some new aspects of the well-known relation between month of birth and incidence of physical and mental handicaps, a relation that already had the attention of the ancient Babylonians and Egyptians (Chapter IV).

Moreover, using the 'overripeness concept' an effort was made to obtain a clearer insight into the interconnection between the various phenotypes commonly known as the Bonnevie-Ullrich-Turner spectrum (Chapters V and VI).

Finally, a set of criteria was formulated which a given congenital abnormality has to meet in order to make overripeness ovopathy acceptable as its possible aetiology. By the use of these criteria it was made plausible that overripeness ovopathy might be a causal moment in Down's syndrome and in several other developmental anomalies (Chapter VII). Again, this needs further confirmation, which can only be obtained by careful interrogation concerning the circumstances around the time of conception.

If it is true that an 'overripe' gamete is, under certain conditions, still capable of participating in the process of fertilization, it is conceivable that the resulting conceptus differs progressively from the normal, in accordance with the degree of overripeness. If this assumption should be valid many variants of human phenomenology and phenotypology could be viewed through other glasses. Therefore, from the nosological point of view the overripeness concept may have its usefulness, both for 'lumpers' and 'splitters' as McKusick calls them. The former it may enable to bring a variety of syndromes, hitherto considered to be separate entities, under a common denominator. The latter may use it as a tool to distinguish, within a given syndrome, between abnormalities caused by overripeness ovopathy and those caused by genetic or peristatic factors.

Far more important, however, are the implications of this concept for everyday medical practice.

First of all the possibility it offers of excluding genetic factors, may considerably lighten the emotional burden borne by parents of congenitally handicapped children.

Secondly, further study of the pathology of conception may result in improvements both in the field of eugenic counselling and in that of family-planning. There are reasons to suppose that the first cautious steps humanity has taken in the latter area have not been entirely successful.

At this point it may be desirable to explain something of the background of this thesis. The process of formation of ideas it contains is reflected in a series of seven articles, presented in chronological sequence. Though they were written in the quiet of the study, they were conceived, and ripened in the daily contacts with patients and their parents, in a centre for observation and treatment of the mentally retarded. The author thinks himself fortunate in having found in *Huize 'Maria Roepaan'* the right climate for this enterprise. The Board of this Foundation deserves both gratitude and praise for its ever-stimulating approach, which has already resulted in a fair number of scientific publications by various staff members.

One of the implications of an investigation of this kind is that it involves constant crossing of boundaries between various disciplines: general biology, teratology, genetics, gynaecology, neuropsychiatry and sexuology, to name the most important. Obviously, this cannot be the work of one person alone, if he does not want to risk making the gravest errors. Therefore, the author is much obliged to countless research-workers past and present, who, often unknowingly, helped him with their data. They collected a great many facts which may have seemed sometimes rather unimportant at the time of publication. The development of the concept of overripeness ovopathy as a working hypothesis for the explanation of certain forms of congenital aberrations, however, would have been unthinkable without their investigations, which often bear witness to great inspiration and perseverance. In his turn the author hopes to have contributed a stimulus for further exploration into the causes of mental retardation and congenital malformations, a field of interest to all who have dedicated themselves to the study of and care for damaged human beings.

It is impossible to mention everyone who in some way or other assisted me at the realization of this thesis. Many of them I already thanked in the acknowledgements following the various articles. Particularly I wish to express my sincere thanks to the parents of the patients. The many conversations they granted me I always experienced as an enrichment.

The nursing staff of *Huize 'Maria Roepaan'* and all others who occupy themselves with the daily care in the Institute, may rest assured of my deep esteem for their devotion.

Drs. G. van der Most, my predecessor as medical director of the Institute, and Dr. P. J. Waardenburg, former Lecturer in Medical Genetics at the University of Leiden, not only have welcomed this study project, but stimulated me and often assisted in finding the right formulations. Others have watched it with wisdom and devotion, contributing especially with critical remarks and suggestions for textual improvements. The first place among those is undoubtedly due to my promotor, Dr. T. D. Stahlie, Professor of Paediatrics at the Free University of Amsterdam, who has contributed much to accomplish this study. His readiness to think with me so intensively deserves my great and lasting gratitude.

Last but not least, I gladly mention my wife, who kindly and patiently assisted me in shaping and re-shaping the numerous versions of the manuscripts on the typewriter. Although reserved and critical with regard to the contents of this thesis, hovering between doubt and personal feelings, I found her always at my side.

Ottersum, August 1971.

Realization of this study has been made possible by the support of the *Stichting 'Sterken Helpen Zwakken'*.

CHAPTER I

CONSIDERATIONS ON THE AETIOLOGY OF GOLDENHAR'S SYNDROME AND RELATED CONGENITAL DYSPLASIAS INCLUDING CHROMOSOMAL ABERRATIONS

BY

P. H. JONGBLOET**

Aim of this article

1. Tp demonstrate the connection between overripeness of the human egg cell and the occurrence of Goldenhar's syndrome (epibulbar dermoids, prae-auricular appendages, congenital aural fistula and vertebral dysplasias).

2. To show that this overripeness of the cytoplasm can also explain the origin of syndromes related to Goldenhar's syndrome. These syndromes generally arise sporadically, vary a lot in expression and form together one group.

3. To show that the occurrence of chromosomal disturbances, both numerical and structural, can be explained by the overripeness theory.

INTRODUCTION

Postovulatory or intratubal overripeness

Overripeness of the egg is not a new idea, having been introduced by PFLÜGER in 1882. By this term he meant ovulated eggs which remained longer than normal in the genital tract before being fertilized. Such eggs show degenerative changes, which finally makes further development impossible, causing them to die. The teratogenic effect of aging on egg cells before fertilization was thoroughly investigated by WITSCHI (1952). Frog's eggs, having been observed becoming gradually overripe, were inseminated artificially and either failed to be fertilized or, if penetrated by a spermatozoön, developed abnormally. Indeed, aging eggs of amphibia gradually lose their vitality. Eggs that are affected slightly by the aging process show only transitory retardations in the rate of development, but overripe eggs may not develop beyond the earliest cleavage stages. BLANDAU (1954) listed some of the

---

* The contents of this paper were presented at the meeting of the Flemish Pediatric Association in Antwerp on 21 September 1968.
** „Huize Maria Roepaan", Institute for mental defectives, Medical Director: G. VAN DER Most, Ottersum (L.) The Netherlands.

developmental abnormalities encountered as the result of overripeness of the eggs in amphibians as follows:

1. tendency to produce axial duplications, especially in the regions of the head. These may take the form of twins, either of equal size and normal appearance, or of unequal dimensions and consisting primarily of teratomatous swellings;
2. polymelia and polydactyly;
3. deficiencies in organogenesis leading in particular to acephaly and microcephaly;
4. failure of the normal differentiation of various tissues and organ systems.

Many investigations in fish and also in mammals pointed in the same direction, except that overripeness occurred even earlier in the latter. BLANDAU (1954) saw that in rats delay of fertilization by 9 to 12 hours after ovulation resulted in non-penetration of 30 % of the eggs by spermatozoa and that more than 40 % of the eggs showed abnormalities even during the pronucleus stage, that is before the first cell division. In only 4 % of the rats did implantation occur.

WITSCHI and LAGUENS (1963) investigated the chromosomes of misformed amphibian embryos obtained by fertilization of aged eggs. They found: a. trisomies and monosomies (non-disjunction), b. haploidy and polyploidy (disturbances in the second meiotic division or polyspermy), c. mosaics, with both two and three clones (disturbances in the first or one of the following cleavage divisions), d. embryos without chromosomal aberrations. They put great emphasis on the embryos described under d, where no chromosomal aberrations were found. In their opinion this indicates that these abnormalities could arise from the teratogenic effect of overripeness. The chromosomal aberrations described under a, b and c could be a consequence of the biochemical or physical changes in the cytoplasm of the egg cell.

SHAVER and CARR (1967) and AUSTIN (1967) carried out similar chromosomal investigations in the rabbit. They, too, observed a rise in the number of abnormalities after delayed fertilization. AUSTIN also investigated the fate of the eggs remaining in the female tract of the rabbit without being fertilized. Three hours after ovulation the chromosomes were still regularly spaced on the equatorial plate of the spindle. After seven hours, however, there was a visible disturbance in more than half, the chromosomes were dispersed and one, two or even three had separated from the group.

Preovulatory or intrafollicular overripeness
Experiments concerning intrafollicular or preovulatory overripeness have been carried out only very recently. MIKAMO (1968) observed in Xenopus

that a great number of intrafollicularly aged eggs were either already dead when spawned, or could not be fertilized, and where this was possible they developed gross abnormalities during the cleavage divisions, gastrulation and neurulation. *He observed acephaly, microcephaly, cyclopy, lateral and dorsoventral flexion and oedema. Most of these embryos died, but some with symptoms such as microcephaly, scoliosis, polymelia or oligomelia survived and developed further.* On microscopic examination it was found that *both ovular components, cytoplasm and nucleus, were affected.* Here, too, one or more tetrads or dyads left the metaphase plate due to poor functioning of one or more spindle fibres. Desintegration of the cytoplasm makes nondisjunction an understandable phenomenon. FUGO and BUTCHER (1966, 1967) investigated intrafollicular overripeness in mammals. In rats they observed a sharp rise of zygotes developing abnormally from the start. If development was allowed to proceed and the embryos could be investigated for chromosomal deviations, again an increase of monosomics, trisomics, polyploids and mosaics was noted.

In conclusion we may say that experiments with amphibians and mammals have proved that both preovulatory and postovulatory overripeness of the egg have desastrous effects on cyto- and caryoplasm. This can have the following consequences: impossibility of fertilization, chromosomal deviations and also developmental disturbances that may or may not cause intrauterine death.

Overripeness in humans
There are reasons to believe that overripeness in man occurs more frequently than in animals. In some animals such as the rabbit, ovulation is induced by coitus, so that the eggs can be fertilized within two or three hours. Moreover, heat in mammals indicates that the egg cells in the ovary are ripe. Heat is caused by folliculine present in the Graafian follicles. As a consequence, syngamy is then at its best or, in other words, neither spermcell nor ovum remains long in the female genitals before fertilization. This is not the case in man. The ovulation period can only be determined by meticulous observation and *coitus is not confined to the fertile period, but can nearly always take place. This stimulates the attractiveness of both partners, although it seems possible that man has had to pay for this advance in evolution by an increase of congenital malformations. Thus the chances rise that the gametes are overripe and that syngamy occurs after the optimal period.*

Experiments in man are impossible, but the problem can be approached indirectly.

HERTIG, ROCK and ADAMS (1956) investigated 34 human zygotes from healthy fertile women in their early development, that is from their two-cell stage until the 17th day. They observed that 21 zygotes developed normally,

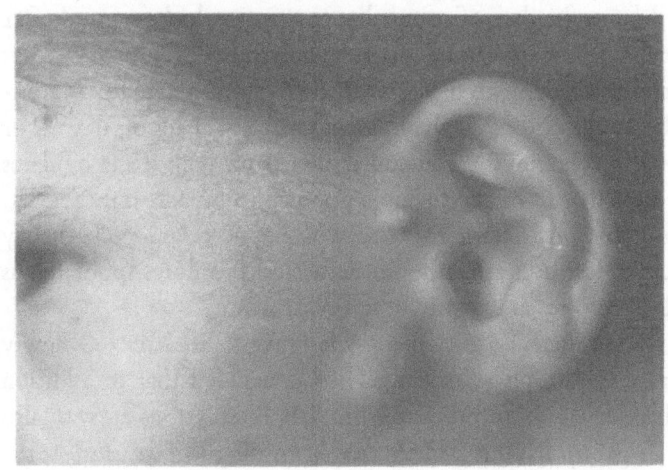

Fig. 1

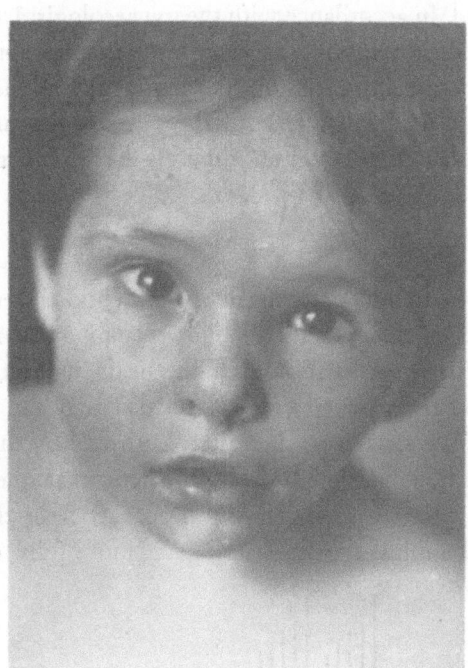

Fig. 2

while 13 proved to be abnormal. In the majority of these (10 out of 13) it could be calculated from the date of coitus that conception had occurred after the 15th day. In the majority (16 out of 20) of the normally developing zygotes this had taken place before the 15th day. HERTIG (1967) returned to this investigation and postulated as follows: if the human female ovulates on day 14 or before, her chances of producing a good conceptus are 92.3 %; if she ovulates on day 15 or later her chances of producing a good conceptus are only 42.8 %.

Between 1961 and 1963 IFFY came forward with his post-mid-cycle theory according to which conception after the fertile period promotes spontaneous abortions, as well as ectopic and pathologic pregnancies.

The findings of BATTAGLIA et al. (1966), who investigated 68.368 newly borns in Baltimore city, are also relevant. They concluded that in addition to a group of children with intrauterine growth retardation, it was also possible to discern a group having a birth weight too high in relation to the duration of the already too short pregnancy. This was shown to be a ,,high-risk" group with a mortality rate 5 times the normal (50.9/1000 and 10.9/1000). One of the possible explanations for this finding was that the too-short pregnancy was really a miscalculation, as 20 % of women during their first month of pregnancy show some form of bleeding which is wrongly interpreted as a menstrual period. In accordance with the gynaecologist IFFY (1962), mentioned above, it would be tempting to choose for this possibility. The ,,high-risk" then would not be due to the bleeding itself, as the authors assume, but would rather be a consequence of the overripeness of the egg as late conception and implantation could not suppress the next menstruation hormonally.

CASE HISTORY

The patient, a girl (figure 1 and 2), was born as sixth child eleven months after the fifth child. The parents practised family planning by means of periodic abstinence. The first menstruation after the birth of the fifth child lasted abnormally long and the parents were certain that they did not have intercourse during the 16 successive days thereafter. Surprised by the absence of the following menstruation, it soon became apparent that the mother was again pregnant. More information is given in another article by this author where the anamnestic and clinical symptomatology is more fully discussed.

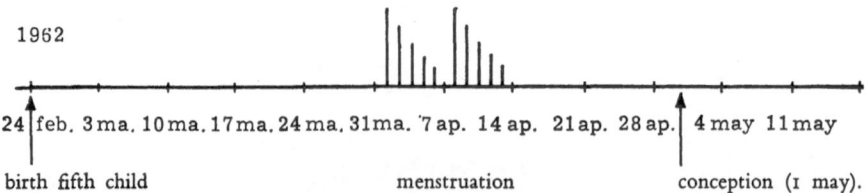

1962

24 | feb. 3 ma. 10 ma. 17 ma. 24 ma. 31 ma. 7 ap. 14 ap. 21 ap. 28 ap. | 4 may 11 may

birth fifth child   menstruation   conception (1 may).

The pregnancy progressed normally except for a slight bleeding around the 5th month, for which the mother spent some days in bed. Towards the end, however, she had many complaints in connection with hydramnios. The mother was 35 and the father 37 years old.

After the child was born, abnormalities were noted concerning eyes, ears and neck. When the patient was 4 years old she was taken into our institute as it was not possible to keep her at home any longer. The mother subsequently had two spontaneous miscarriages, one of which when 39 years old. Of this particular one it is known that conception could only have occurred on the 26th day after menstruation. The parents still practised periodic abstinence. No cases of mental retardation or congenital abnormalities were recorded in this family, apart from one case of meningomyelocele in the grandmother's family on the mother's side.

CLINICAL DATA

The patient showed stunted growth, dermoids on both eyes, starting from the limbus corneae, and brevi-torticollis as a result of Klippel-Feil vertebral abnormalities. Further there exists left hemifacial hypoplasia and paresis, retractio bulbi, auricular appendages and blind-ending fistulas. Audiological tests showed serious loss of air conduction, predominantly on the left side. Extensive biochemical and cytogenetical investigations showed no abnormalities. Dermatoglyphic investigation showed a disturbance in the interdigital IV: in the right hand palm a superfluous triradius and in the left a double loop were noted. On the finger tips nine ulnary loops and a „tented-arch" are present. Psychological tests (Stutsman IQ = 77) show her to be mentally retarded, but educable.

DISCUSSION

The etiological connection between overripeness of the egg cell and the occurrence of Goldenhar's syndrome can be argued as follows.

First there are casuistic arguments:

a. It may be assumed on good grounds that in the mother concerned ovulation occurred too late, and that this is a case of intrafollicular and possibly intratubal overripeness. The previous menstruation had been extremely prolonged and it is known that the normal hormonal balance equilibrates itself less easily after pregnancy. In addition the mother was already 35 years old. The spontaneous bleeding in the 5th month of pregnancy may have indicated the abnormality of the foetus with a tendency towards abortion.

b. The discordant occurrence of Goldenhar's syndrome in monovular twins as mentioned by BOCK (1951). Also NAROG (1926) and GOLDENHAR himself (1952) described discordant occurrence without mentioning, however, whether this concerned monovular or binovular twins. We will return to this aspect of discordance in one-egg twins, as this is a very intriguing phenomenon in Goldenhar's and other syndromes.

c. Finally, ZARFL's communication (1935) proved to be of great significance. He described a child that after a tubal pregnancy was born alive by means of laparatomy and showed the typical abnormalities found in the oculo-auriculo-vertebral syndrome. This communication is important, since it fits in with IFFY's idea, postulating that tubal pregnancies are due to late fertilization.

Secondly, no other good reasons have been brought forward pointing to a different etiology. Furthermore, the abnormalities found in Goldenhar's syndrome are comparable to those found in amphibia after preovulatory (MIKAMO) and postovulatory (WITSCHI) overripeness, such as a tendency to give rise to identical twins, sometimes of normal appearance but sometimes of unequal size; eventually a tendency towards polydactyly, deficiencies in organogenesis and inadequate differentiation of various tissues and organ systems (gill arches and facies).

Moreover, there are numerous transitions to other syndromes and congenital malformations, which are sometimes impossible to differentiate diagnostically. For instance, our patient could be taken for a case of Goldenhar's syndrome, but also for one of hemifacial microsomy, a Wildervanck's syndrome (1960 and 1963), an oculo-vertebral syndrome, and many others.

The sporadic occurrence of Goldenhar's syndrome also needs attention. Only one family is known (SARAUX, 1963) with two girls showing ear and eye abnormalities analogous to those occurring in Goldenhar's syndrome. In this case, however, the dermoids did not seem to start from the limbus corneae. Partly based on this family, the oculo-auriculo-vertebral syndrome was listed by McKUSICK as an autosomal recessive disease. We feel, however, that this unique case could be explained by endocrinological or other factors causing delayed ovulation. In this way, intrafollicular overripeness could repeat itself. The complicated interplay between heredity and the overripeness problem might then be a decisive factor for a deviation in a certain direction. Another possibility is that in this family we are concerned with a genocopy.

Finally, variation in intelligence and a variable effect on the central nervous system are more easily explained by the overripeness theory. GORLIN notes that 10 % of those affected by Goldenhar's syndrome are retarded. The degree to which the central nervous system is affected could be decisive here.

In conclusion therefore, we may postulate the following hypothesis:

1. *Goldenhar's syndrome or the oculo-auriculo-vertebral syndrome is due to over-ripeness of the egg.*

The second aim of our paper is to show *that this overripeness theory can explain the origin of many related syndromes.*

As mentioned previously, Goldenhar's syndrome is hard to delimit. In addition to the typical abnormalities affecting eyes, ears and vertebrae, less marked deviations of eyes, mouth, ribs and central nervous system have been noted. Consequently it is difficult to distinguish Goldenhar's syndrome from the hemifacial microsomy, the retractio-bulbi syndrome (Stilling-Duane-Türck), the „first-arch" syndrome (McKenzie), the mandibulofacial dysostosis (Nager and De Reynier) and the otomandibular dysostosis (François-Haustrate). We tend to include Klippel-Feil's syndrome types 1 and III, the cervico-oculo-acusticus syndrome (Wildervanck), the oculo-vertebral syndrome (Weyers-Thier), the status dysrhaphicus (Bremer) and the combination of symptoms recently reported by Say and Gerald (1968) (polydactyly, imperforate anus and vertebral abnormalities), along with less sharply defined vertebral abnormalities. The dyscraniopygophalangy or „Typus Rostockiensis" (Bartholin-Ullrich-Feichtiger) also seems related. The connections between Goldenhar's syndrome and dysplasias of the central nervous system are illustrated in the case of Hoffmann-Egg and Velissaro-poulos (1953) where an ocular dermoid-lipoid and a meningoencephalocele occurred together. As early as 1886, Picqué reported that this association was quite frequently found. In other cases (Cohen 1923 and Inoue 1938) auricular appendages and dermolipoids are coupled with a cleft palate, hare lip and wolf snout.

In this whole group of abnormalities, where sometimes dermolipoids or auricular appendages, and at other times vertebral abnormalities, dysplasias of the central nervous system or polydactyly dominate, some general characteristics can be discovered.

1. All these dysmorphies, including Goldenhar's syndrome, occur sporadically.
2. They are often found concordantly, but more often discordantly, in one-egg twins (Record and McKeown 1950; Cameron et al. 1968; Yen and McMahon 1968). The analogy with Witschi's findings of duplications as a result of overripeness of the egg in amphibians must be stressed here.
3. Further, the degree of intellectual handicap varies considerably among the victims of these dysplasias. The brain can be minimally, but also seriously, affected in the same syndrome.
4. Finally, hydramnios during pregnancy is of frequent occurrence (Bucking-ham, 1960). The mother concerned also had unexplained hydramnios. Sayegh (1963) saw it in 100 % of his cases of anencephaly.

It is interesting to trace the analogy between these dysplasias and the abnormalities of human embryos obtained from spontaneous and induced abortions.

NISHIMURA et al. (1966) investigated 3.402 human embryos between 3 and 4 weeks old, which had been aborted for social reasons. Of these 38 (1.12 %) were misformed. Among other abnormalities exencephaly, myeloschisis and cyclopy were encountered. Similar abnormalities are known in spontaneous abortions (POLAND, 1968). The last miscarriage of the mother of our patient gives rise to the suspicion that this was caused by pre- or postovulatory overripeness in a case of late fertilization of the egg. We know that in this case coitus took place only on the 26th day.

From studies concerning the frequency of dysplasias of the central nervous system in various ethnic groups (NAGGAN and McMAHON, 1967; COLLMAN and STOLLER, 1968) great differences became apparent. In Irish families the frequency of anencephaly and spina bifida cystica was 2.79/1000 and in Jewish families only 0.77/1000. These authors believe that the occurrence of these diseases cannot be explained by the usual hereditary theories, but that environmental factors must play a part. In this connection Cross's remark (1968) needs full attention. On the one hand he connects the more frequent occurrence of these abnormalities in Irish (Roman Catholic) families with the application of periodic abstinence. In Jewish families on the other hand the „Niddah" is applied, demanding abstinence until the 11th day. Therewith the chance that fertilization takes place shortly after ovulation rises. Moreover, in his experience (1961) fertility rose and congenital malformations decreased in number when couples abstained until the 11th day of the cycle. LANMAN (1968) too, expected on the basis of animal experiments a rise in the number of congenital malformations among couples applying periodic abstinence; specific cases, however, were not known to him.

We conclude with the following hypotheses:

II. *The mainly sporadically occurring congenital dysplasias are related to each other and can be considered as one group.* We would like to include in this group Goldenhar's syndrome, Wildervanck's syndrome, status dysrhaphicus, the status Bonnevie-Ullrich, the spina bifida cystica and many others. Further delimitation is still hardly possible.

III. *The origin of these sporadically occurring phenomena and their clinical variability are better explained by the overripeness theory than by other etiologies, such as the hereditary processes.* It is also possible that the reverse process, namely unripeness of the egg due to early ovulation, too, leads to pathology. The same is true of abnormalities in the sperm. Little is known of both these phenomena, even in animals.

IV. *The severity of the diseases can vary from mild to very serious according to the degree of cytoplasmatic disturbance.*

v. *It is probable that in this manner phenocopies arise of existing genetical entities,* such as the retractio-bulbi syndrome, that in 10 % of the cases is inherited in an autosomal dominant manner (FRANÇOIS 1968).

vi. *A considerable proportion of spontaneous abortions could be due to the overripeness phenomenon of the egg cell.*

* * *

The third aim of this article is to postulate that *chromosomal aberrations can also arise in this way.*

First of all we should like to point out that not only the number of chromosomal aberrations, but also that of cases of anencephaly and spina bifida cystica rises with the age of the mother. Analogous processes seem possible. GERMAN (1968) showed statistically that the occurrence of mongolism in the progeny of older women is more strongly correlated with the number of years of marriage than with the age of the mother. The lowered frequency of intercourse, along with the rising number of years of marriage, increases the chance of fertilization of an overripe egg cell, because the chances then are smaller that the ovum will be fertilized immediately after ovulation. PENROSE and BERG (1968) carried out a similar investigation on the duration of marriage of the parents of 988 mongoloid children, using other mentally deficient children as controls but could not confirm GERMAN's results, although they did not reject his hypothesis. In this controversy PENROSE and BERG failed to realise that other types of mental deficiency can also originate from the overripening process, as we argued above. For this reason we consider it wrong to take mentally deficient children as a control group.

More important still are the results of chromosomal investigations in spontaneous abortion (CARR 1967 and many others), one-egg twins (NIELSEN 1967) and mentally deficient children (VAN GELDEREN 1967), because these findings show a remarkable similarity with the data of experimental animal research into intrafollicular or intratubal overripeness. We cannot go more deeply into this here, but special note should be made of the high frequency of triploids in mola hydatidosa as reported by ATKIN and KLINGER (1962), MAKINO et al. (1964), SZULMAN (1965), and BOUÉ et al. (1967). This type of pathologic pregnancy is, according to IFFY (1962), clearly connected with delayed fertilization; the menstruation which could not be suppressed, washes away the recently implanted embryo, so that the trophoblast develops on its own. It is also known that the chance of mola hydatidosa rises with the age of the mother. Moreover, it should be pointed out that there is an increase in chromosomal aberrations in spontaneous abortions (1/250 in normal births and 1/4 in spontaneous abortions). These findings have often been confirmed. Why many monosomies of the sex chromosomes and trisomies of the small autosomes are aborted, is not clear as they are quite compatible with normal intrauterine stay. This phenomenon might indicate that these chromosomal disturbances are only the result of a more fundamental disturbance that is responsible for both serious malformations and spontaneous abortion.

Until recently animal research was usually limited to numerical deviations caused by disturbances in syngamy, non-disjunction occurring during meiosis or during the first or following cleavage divisions. MIKAMO (1968) however, noticed in the case of extreme overripeness of amphibian eggs, fracturing of the chromosomes, so that structural aberrations could be explained as well by the overripeness theory. We have indications that this phenomenon also occurs in man.

That cytoplasmatic disturbances in the overripe egg cell can give rise to both congenital abnormalities and chromosomal aberrations can be deduced from the fact that they may occur combined. For instance, in our institute we have two patients with Klippel-Feil vertebral anomalies, one combined with Down's syndrome and the other with Turner's syndrome. Both patients are even more mentally retarded than usual. In our opinion their degree of mental retardation is not primarily caused by the trisomy 21 or the XO-pattern, respectively, but by the extent to which the nervous system is affected by the cytoplasmatic disturbances of the egg cell, analogous to the case of dysplasias of the central nervous system without chromosomal aberrations. We are also convinced that the retractio-bulbi syndrome, sometimes occurring in conjunction with status Bonnevie-Ullrich, is caused in fact by a disturbance in the cytoplasm. This then would be responsible for both the dysmorphy and the chromosomal anomaly. If our hypothesis is correct, then the retractio-bulbi syndrome should also occur in conjunction with other chromosomal aberrations such as mongolism. This indeed proves to be the case, since LOESCH-MDZEWSKA (1968) found, during a neurological investigation of 123 mongoloid patients, two patients where Down's syndrome was combined with Horner's syndrome. The very high percentages of both pupillary irregularity (up to 75 %) and convergent squint (about 25 %) indicate the presence of frustrated forms of the Stilling-Duane-Türck syndrome in mongoloid patients. Perhaps too the „male Turner" syndrome and status Bonnevie-Ullrich without chromosomal aberrations are easier to understand in this way. The same reasoning may be applied to the analysis of dermatoglyphic patterns which have been found to vary so much in the numerous clinical syndromes with or without chromosomal aberrations.

We conclude with two hypotheses:

VII. *Chromosomal aberrations can be caused by overripeness of the egg cell.*
VIII. *A cytoplasmatic disturbance may lead to congenital dysplasias associated with chromosomal anomalies.*

The question still remains, however, whether reverse phenomena, such as „unripeness of the egg cell" due to too early ovulation, or aging of the male gamete, may cause similar deviations. We are under the impression that in the former phenomenon this is indeed the case.

* * *

CONCLUSION

From experimental findings in animals it might be expected that also in man pre- and postovulatory overripeness can lead to pathologic conditions. Intercourse in man is not confined to certain periods as is the case with animals. This progress in partnership also has a drawback, since conception now becomes possible after the optimal period for fertilization. Should fertilization occur at a too late stage, disturbances in the cytoplasm of the ovum, the zygote and the first blastomeres may arise. As is the case in animals it is reasonable to suppose that the egg cell, as a result of overripeness, cannot be fertilized or degenerates before implantation. If affected to a lesser degree, then abnormalities may develop which either result in intrauterine death or are compatible with intrauterine life. This last group will show much variation since endogenous and other exogenous factors also play a part.

In addition to and independently of the phenomena mentioned here, numerical and possibly also structural chromosomal aberrations may arise during syngamy, the meiosis or the first cleavage divisions. This may promote degeneration of the embryo. Evidently known factors such as an increased chance for nondisjunction in older mothers and in the case of virus infections (virus hepatitis) are not in contradiction with the explanation offered.

The above is no more than a set of working hypotheses which, however, can be supported by important arguments. They should be further verified, supported and expanded by continued research in animals and by continued accurate observations of human pathology. Here it seems the right place to emphasize that general practitioners, gynaecologists and paediatricians, when confronted with pathology in the human progeny, should pay particular attention to all information concerning the moment of conception. Much patience on the doctor's part and a certain amount of intelligence of the couples concerned will be necessary. The little knowledge available at present already leads one to question the apparent harmlessness of periodic abstinence, without basal-body-temperature control, as a means of birth control; this holds especially true for older and irregularly ovulating women.

SUMMARY

The parents of a girl, with all symptoms of the oculo-auriculo-vertebral dysplasia or GOLDENHAR's syndrome, practised periodic abstinence. The new pregnancy could only be explained by assuming that the ovulation occurred too late. Therefore, intrafollicular and possibly intratubal overripeness of the ovum was likely.

The literature on overripeness of the ovum in animals is reviewed. Analogical findings in human pathology were collected.

The etiology of GOLDENHAR's syndrome and related congenital malformations is discussed. In this connection overripeness of the ovum is postulated. Accepting this theory of overripeness a new unitary conception about the origin of a great number of dysplasias develops, whereby the fluent transition and the mainly sporadic appearance becomes more intelligible. The hypothesis that chromosomal anomalies may also originate through overripeness, can be defended by means of convincing arguments.

The present author emphasizes the necessity of collecting more accurate information about the time of conception of normal and abnormal offspring. In view of these facts it is possible that periodic abstinence, without basal-body-temperature control, may endanger the health of human progeny as it favours the odds of fertilization of an overripe egg.

SAMENVATTING

Ondanks periodieke onthouding der ouders, ontstond een ongewenste zwangerschap waaruit een meisje werd geboren dat alle symptomen vertoonde van het oculo-auriculo-vertebrale syndroom van GOLDENHAR. Deze zwangerschap kon alleen worden verklaard door aan te nemen dat de ovulatie te laat was opgetreden waardoor intrafolliculaire en mogelijk ook intratubaire overrijping van de eicel bestond.

De literatuur over de overrijping van het ovum bij dieren werd nagegaan. Analoge bevindingen uit de menselijke pathologie werden verzameld.

De etiologie van het syndroom van GOLDENHAR en andere congenitale misvormingen wordt ter discussie gesteld. In dit verband wordt overrijping van de eicel gepostuleerd. Neemt men deze overrijpingstheorie aan, dan ontstaat een eenheidsconcept betreffende een groot aantal dysplasieën, waardoor de vloeiende overgangen en het hoofdzakelijk sporadisch voorkomen ervan zich beter laten verklaren. Dat ook chromosomale stoornissen bij de mens mede door overrijping kunnen ontstaan, wordt aan de hand van diverse argumenten verdedigd.

Er wordt aangedrongen op het verzamelen van meer nauwkeurige informatie over de conceptietijd van normale en abnormale progenituur. Zoals de feiten zich nu voordoen, kan men zich niet onttrekken aan de indruk dat periodieke onthouding zonder temperatuurscontrole gevaren kan meebrengen voor de menselijke progenituur, daar deze de kansen op bevruchting van een overrijpe eicel bevordert.

P.S. To test these hypotheses we have investigated more systematically the day of conception of our recent patients. Of eight couples with a child with Down's syndrome four assured us that these children were conceived despite application of periodic abstinence. In addition, periodic abstinence was also involved in a case of structural chromosomal aberration, a case of male Turner syndrome and six cases of dyscephalia, two of which were clearly asymmetric and thus related to Goldenhar's syndrome. These cases will be discussed in greater detail elsewhere.

LITERATURE

ATKIN, N. B. and H. P. KLINGER: The superfemale mole, Lancet 2: 727, 1962.
AUSTIN, C. R.: Chromosome deterioration in ageing eggs of the rabbit, Nature 213: 1018, 1967.
BATTAGLIA, F. C., T. M. FRAZIER and A. E. HELLEGERS: Birth weight, gestational age, and pregnancy outcome, with special reference to high birth weight-low gestational age infant, Pediatrics 37: 417, 1966.
BLANDAU, R. J.: The effects on development when eggs and sperm are aged before fertilization, Ann. N.Y. Acad. Sci. 57:526, 1954.
BOCK, R. H.: Ein Fall von epibulbarem Dermolipom mit Missbildungen einer Gesichtshälfte, Diskordantes Vorkommen bei einem eineiigen Zwillingspaar, Ophthalmologica 122: 86, 1951.
BOUÉ, J. G., A. BOUÉ and P. LAZAR: Les aberrations chromosomiques dans les avortements, Ann. Génét. 10: 179, 1967.
BUCKINGHAM, J. C., T. W. McELIN, V. M. BOWERS and J. McVAY: A clinical study of hydramnios, Obst. and Gynec. 15: 652, 1960.
BUTCHER, R. L. and N. W. FUGO: Overripeness and the mammalian ova. II. Delayed ovulation and chromosome anomalies, Fertil and Steril. 18: 297, 1967.
CAMERON, A. H., J. H. EDWARDS, R. DEROM, M. THIERY and R. BOELAERT: The value of twin surveys in the study of malformations, communication in Ghent by R. Derom on 19.10.1968.
CARR, D. H.: Chromosome anomalies as a cause of spontaneous abortion. Amer. J. Obstet. Gynec. 97: 283, 1967.
COHEN, C.: Dermoid of conjunctiva, Med. J. Aust. 2: 360, 1924, cited by Goldenhar (1952).
COLLMANN, R. D. and A. STOLLER: The occurrence of anencephalus in the state of Victoria, Australia, J. ment. Defic. Res. 12: 22, 1968.
CROSS, R. G.: Prevention of anencephaly and foetal abnormalities, Lancet 2: 1124, 1961.
CROSS, R. G.: Anencephalus and spina bifida, Brit. Med. J. 3: 253, 1968.
FRANÇOIS, J.· Congenitale ophthalmoplegieën, communication in Antwerp on 29.9.1968.

Fugo, N. W. and R. L. Butcher: Overripeness and the mammalian ova. I. Overripeness and early embryonic development, Fertil. and Steril. 17: 804, 1966.

Gelderen, H. H. van, A. Schaberg and J. L. J. Gaillard et al.: Een onderzoek naar chromosomale afwijkingen bij zwakzinnige niet mongoloïde kinderen, Maandschr. Kindergeneesk. 35: 141, 1967.

German, J.: Mongolism, delayed fertilization and human sexual behavior, Nature 217: 516, 1968.

Goldenhar, M.: Associations des malformations de l'oeil et de l'oreille en particulier le syndrome dermoïde épibulbaire-appendices auriculaires- fistula auris congenita et ses relations avec la dysostose mandibulo-faciale, J. Génét. hum. 1: 243, 1952.

Hertig, A. T., J. Rock and E. C. Adams: A description of 34 human ova within the first 17 days of development, Amer. J. Anat. 98: 435, 1956.

Hertig, A. T.: Human trophoblast: normal and abnormal, Amer. J. clin. Path. 47: 249, 1967.

Hoffmann-Egg, L., P. Velissaropoulos, Malformations oculo-auriculaires et leur relations avec la dysostose mandibulo-faciale, Ann. Oculist. (Paris) 186: 155, 1953.

Iffy, L.: Contribution to the aetiology of ectopic pregnancy, J. Obstet. Gynaec. Brit. cwlth. 68: 441, 1961.

Iffy, L. and P. Kerner: The aetiology of early abortion, J. Obstet. Gynaec. Brit. cwlth. 69: 598, 1962.

Iffy, L.: Contribution to the aetiology of hydatidiform mole, Ann. Chir. Gynaec. Fenn. 51: 428, 1962.

Iffy, L.: The time of conception in pathological gestations, Proc. roy. Soc. Med. 56: 1098, 1963.

Iffy, L.: The role of premenstrual, post-midcycle conception in the aetiology of ectopic gestation, J. Obstet. Gynaec. Brit. cwlth. 70: 996, 1963.

Inoue, M.: Ein seltener Fall von beiderseits symmetrischem Limbus-dermoid mit Hasenscharte und Wofsrachen, Zbl. f. ges. Ophthal. 42: 303, 1939.

Jongbloet, P. H.: cited in the editorial of Katholiek Artsenblad 47: 314, 1968.

Jongbloet, P. H.: Overrijpheid van het ovum. Beschouwingen over de etiologie van het syndroom van Goldenhar en aanverwante congenitale dysplasieën, Ned. T. Geneesk. 113: 653, 1969. Ibidem 113: 1215, 1969.

Lanman, J. T.: Delays during reproduction and their effects on the embryo and fetus. 2. Aging of eggs, New Engl. J. Med. 278: 1047, 1968.

Loesch-Mdzewska, Danuta: Some aspects of the neurology of Down's Syndrome, J. Ment. Defic. Res. 12: 237, 1968.

Makino, S., M. S. Sasaki and T. Fukuschima: Triploid chromosome constitution in human chorionic lesions, Lancet 2: 1273, 1964.

Mikamo, K.: Intrafollicular overripeness and teratologic development, Cytogenetics 7: 212, 1968.

Mikamo, K.: Mechanism of non-disjunction of meiotic chromosomes and of degeneration of maturation spindles in eggs affected by intrafollicular overripeness, Experientia 24: 75, 1968.

Naggan, L. and B. MacMahon: Ethnic differences in the prevalence of anencephaly and spina bifida in Boston, Massachussetts, New Engl. J. Med. 277: 1119, 1967.

Narog, F.: Bindehaut-Hornhautdermoide beider Augen, Zbl. ges. Ophthal. 15: 707, 1926.

Nielsen, J.: Inheritance in monozygotic twins, Lancet 2: 717, 1967.

Nishimura, H., K. Takano, T. Tanimura, M. Yasuda and T. Uchida: High incidence of several malformations in the early human embryos as compared with infants, Biol. Neonat. 10: 93, 1966.

Penrose, L. S. and J. M. Berg: Mongolism and duration of marriage, Nature 218: 300, 1968.

Picqué, L.: Anomalies de développement et maladies congénitales du globe de l'oeil, 1886, cited by Goldenhar (1952).

Poland, B. J.: Study of developmental anomalies in the spontaneously aborted fetus, Amer. J. Obstet. Gynec. 100: 501, 1968.

Record, R. G. and T. McKeown: Congenital malformations of the central nervous system, Ann. Eugenics 15: 285, 1950.

Saraux, H., J. L. Grignon and P. Dhermy: A propos d'une observation familiale de syndrome de Franceschetti-Goldenhar, Bull. Soc. Ophthal. franç. 63: 705, 1963.

Say, B. and P. S. Gerald: A new polydactyly/imperforate-anus/vertebral anomalies syndrome?, Lancet 2: 688, 1968.

Sayegh, C.: Contribution à l'étude de l'étiologie des malformations congénitales, J. Génét. hum. 12: 91, 1963.

Shaver, E. L. and D. H. Carr: Chromosome abnormalities in rabbit blastocysts following delayed fertilization, J. Reprod. Fertil. 147: 415, 1967.

20

Szulman, A. W.: Chromosomal aberrations in spontaneous human abortions, *New Engl. J. Med.* 27: 811, 1965.

Wildervanck, L. S.: Een cervico-oculo-acusticussyndroom, *Ned. T. Geneesk.* 104: 2601, 1960.

Witschi, E.: Overripeness of the egg as a cause of twinning and teratogenesis, A review. *Cancer Research* 12: 763, 1952.

Witschi, E. and R. Laguens: Chromosomal aberrations in embryos from overripe eggs, *Develop. Biol.* 7: 605, 1963.

Yen, S. and B. MacMahon: Genetics of anencephaly and spina bifida? *Lancet* 2: 623, 1968.

Zarfl, M.: Uber ein lebendes missbildetes Kind nach ausgetragener Eileiterschwangerschaft, *Z. Kinderheilk.* 57: 505, 1935.

I wish to express my thanks to G. van der Most, medical director of the institute „Huize Maria Roepaan", for his stimulation and assistance in this work. I should also like to thank the staff for their collaboration and Mrs. G. A. van der Mey, B.Sc., for translating this paper into English.

CHAPTER II

THE INTRIGUING PHENOMENON OF GAMETOPATHY AND ITS DISASTROUS EFFECTS ON THE HUMAN PROGENY*

BY

P. H. JONGBLOET**, paediatrician

INTRODUCTION

In previous publications (JONGBLOET 1968, 1969) we pointed out that the investigator confronted with mentally retarded human progeny should pay strict attention to the time and circumstances under which fertilization concerned took place. The possibility that overripeness of the ovum is the cause of a number of congenital dysplasias, with or without chromosomal aberrations, was postulated. Classical theories on heredity cannot explain some important facts such as the causes of the increased frequency of congenital aberrations in primiparous women as well as with rising age of the mother. Also the basis of discordant occurrence of such abnormalities in one-egg twins is not understood. All attempts to explain these facts by exogenic factors have failed so far.

The overripeness-of-the-egg phenomenon has been established by means of experimental animal research, both in amphibia and in mammals. The possibility of increased teratogenic action has been shown to exist both in preovulatory or intrafollicular, and in postovulatory or intratubal overripeness (WITSCHI 1952, FUGO and BUTCHER 1966, 1967 and 1969 and MIKAMO 1968).

In this perspective different hypotheses were formulated concerning man's progeny. The fertilization of an overripe egg could lead _1._ to delayed menstruation (due to incomplete implantation), _2._ to spontaneous abortion, _3._ to a nonviable foetus at birth or _4._ to congenital malformations in the newborn, especially dysplasias of the central nervous system. It is with this last group

---

* The contents of this paper were presented at the 3rd International Conference on Congenital Malformations. The Hague, The Netherlands, 7—13 Sept. 1969.

** „Huize Maria Roepaan", Institute for mental defectives; Medical Director: G. VAN DER MOST, Ottersum (L.), The Netherlands.

Maandschr. Kindergeneesk., 37: 261, 1969.

that the staff of an observation centre for the mentally retarded is most often confronted. It is well enough known that in these products of pathological pregnancies there may be numerical or structural chromosomal deviations. It is not yet clear whether certain chromosomal aberrations are responsible for certain congenital malformations. It remains, for instance, unexplained why 39 out of 40 foetuses with the xo configuration die in utero (CARR 1967), while this chromosomal anomaly in itself is compatible with intra- as well as extrauterine life. Neither is there an explanation for the whole spectrum of aberrations between, on the one hand, the male Turner syndrome and, on the other hand, the syndrome of Bonnevie-Ullrich, both with a normal chromosomal pattern, and between these the classical Turner syndrome as a special nuance with its female phenotype and many chromosomal variations. An equally intriguing problem is the occurrence in both Down's syndrome and Turner's syndrome, of isolated congenital aberrations of the eyes (blepharophimosis, macrocornea, ptosis), the ears, the facial skull bones, the vertebrae (Klippel-Feil's anomalies) and the extremities. These anomalies are also found in congenitally degenerative cases in which no chromosomal deviations are present. All these phenomena might be more clearly understood in the light of the overripeness theory, whereby neither the chromosomal nor the congenital deviations are to be looked upon as either cause or effect, but both are the consequence of a common aetiology, namely ovopathy. The occurrence of this phenomenon — (and also of superannuated sperm) — in man is quite likely and even to be expected, since in this species ovulation does neither occur as a reflex after coition as in some animals, nor spontaneously during heat as in other animals. In man coition occurs during the whole menstrual cycle, both before and after ovulation. Thus the probability of fertilization by or of superannuated gametes rises.

To test these hypotheses we have questioned 127 couples about the circumstances and the moments of fertilization of all their pregnancies. On the surface this may seem a difficult task. Some facts however, can be verified, such as a „failure" during the rhythmic method, and pregnancies arising before menstruation had returned after a birth or abortion. Also, the time interval between two successive births and between marriage (first coition) and first birth or (abortion) can be accurately determined.

INVESTIGATION

The information for the investigation was obtained through intensive talks with 127 couples having one or more mentally retarded children, 131 propositi in all. The couples were questioned about methods of contraception, the number of menstrual cycles between pregnancies, the taking of drugs before fertilization and the frequency of sexual intercourse during the period of conception. These data were, as far as possible, also collected for normal progeny. The total number of pregnancies was 633, including 91 cases of abortion. All parents of our patients are Roman Catholics; the age of the propositi was around eight years. In the great majority of cases a mutual trust has grown between the parents and the investigator, so that the parents were prepared to cooperate in the investigation. All parents were questioned two or three times at intervals of several weeks or months, by which means their previous statements could be checked. If there was any doubt about the correctness of the data, they were not included in our statistics. No selection was applied on account of the degree of mental retardation, and all forms of congenital deviations, abortions and mental deficiency were included. In only 9 cases of mental retardation was there a clearly defined post-natal cause; 7 times encephalitis and twice a definite hyperbilirubinemia. We felt obliged to include all these forms since there is a possibility that all kinds of troubles in the newborn, such as underweight, undertemperature, respiratory difficulties with cyanosis etc., are basically due to defective development based on ovopathy. It seemed also reasonable to ask whether post-natal encephalitis (of an infectious or postvaccinal nature) might not be due to a cerebrum already affected in its origin; it is for this reason that we took these cases also into consideration. We want to emphasize that none of the propositi suffered from any known genetic or metabolic disease.

In view of a logical presentation of our findings we divided our data into five main categories.

Categorie I consisted of 35 couples who had applied the rhythmic method as a means of contraception, in spite of which a pregnancy had occurred. In only two cases was the rhythmic method combined with basal temperature control. Couples applying coitus interruptus during the fertile period were not included in this group.

Category I is divided into four groups:

Group I A which is again subdivided into the subgroups A 1 to A 5 depending on the „safe period" used.

Group I B consists of two sets of parents who considered only the first day after menstruation as safe.

Group I C consists of 5 couples wherein pregnancies had occurred immediately after departure from the prescribed or planned rhythmic method.
One should wonder in these cases, however, whether these pregnancies were
not rationalized afterwards and thus looked upon as wanted. MARSHALL (1968)
points out this possibility and groups these under „accidental pregnancy".
Moreover, in four of these cases it seems possible that conception had taken
place before the last menstruation, considering the birth weight and the duration
of the pregnancy, and thus during the period of the applied rhythmic method.
IFFY (1962, 1963, 1968) points out the possibility of premenstrual conception;
if this occurs just before menstruation, bleeding can no longer be suppressed.

Group I D includes 5 couples who stated that the „failure" was due to careless
application of the rhythmic method. In this type of „accidental pregnancy",
the possibility of a low coition frequency during the fertile period should be
considered, thus increasing the chances of fertilization of an overripe egg.

Category II consists of 26 couples in which one or more pregnancies occurred
soon after an abortion, a birth, durante lactatione or after the application of
hormonal steroids.

Group II A includes 18 couples who remembered that a pregnancy had occurred before or after the first menstruation, after an abortion, after a birth or
while nursing. We did not distinguish between those cases where none or
one menstruation had taken place before conception, as the literature concerned shows that the first ovulation may occur before as well as after the
first menstruation.

Group II B includes 13 pregnancies of which the parents could not remember
exactly the time interval between birth or abortion and the next pregnancy,
but where the birth occurred within 365 days after the previous birth or
abortion.

Group II C consists of 2 defective children begotten just after prolonged use
of combined drugs to suppress ovulation.

Category III
The first pregnancy of a woman may be conceived pre- or postnuptially. The
occurrence of a pregnancy immediately after marriage, without premarital
intercourse has, in the framework of this study, a special significance. The
first coition can have taken place after ovulation, thus increasing the chance

of fertilization of an intratubal overripe egg. In addition, irregularity of the menstrual cycle due to stress should be taken into account. Several women found that menstruation in the honeymoon period occurred earlier than expected. Most strikingly it occurred in some cases on the wedding day, naturally an undesirable and unplanned moment. As a cycle shortened in this manner is often followed by a compensatory lengthened one, the possibility of intrafollicular overripeness should also be considered. DÖRING (1967) points out that shifts of the ovulation after a previous irregular cycle are quite common.

Group III D consists of 39 pregnancies where conception occurred within the first or second menstrual cycle after the day of marriage. Couples stating that they had had pre-marital intercourse were not included in this group. 325 days was taken as the extreme time limit between marriage and birth.

Group III E is in a similar way composed of 16 pregnancies, conceived before the wedding-day.

In *category IV* those mothers that had been treated with a barbiturate for epilepsy or nervousness at the time of fertilization were included *(Group F)*. Animal research has shown that these drugs, and also neuroleptica, can delay and even cause suppression of ovulation. Therefore, too, the possibility of intrafollicular overripening must be taken into account.

In *category V* attention was paid to case histories in which some notes concerning the conception seemed important.

In the first four categories children were considered „normal" when the parents were of this opinion and „abnormal" when retardation or objective congenital deviations were present. Abortions were registered separately and grouped together with abnormal pregnancies to compare their frequencies expressed as percentages with the frequencies of normal children. For comparison, each time a group was formed out of all other pregnancies in the same families, while the groups were subdivided in the same manner. These „comparison groups" within the same families have the advantage of cancelling out other common exogenous factors or possible unknown genetic influences.

A statistical evaluation of this material was impossible because the subject of the investigation did not form an aselect population group. The parents were namely selected on having at least one mentally retarded child and on being Roman Catholics. The total number of propositi is given in brackets. Within the various categories investigated we have also calculated the percentages of normal and abnormal progeny without including the number of propositi. This might perhaps give an idea of what occurs as „conceptopathology" in the normal population. Possible errors in this assumption will be discussed later.

Twins were always counted as one pregnancy, normal when both were normal, abnormal when one or both were such. The average maternal age is calculated for all categories, subgroups and comparison groups at conception, not at delivery.

RESULTS
These are presented in tables I and II.

DISCUSSION
I. The highest percentage of disturbed pregnancies was observed with the strictest application of the rhythmic method, in which only the premenstrual phase was observed as safe period (I A 1). It was noticed that this group concerned parents having such strong motives that they had limited cohabitation to only a few days before the expected menstruation for fear of a pregnancy. Here combinations are possible of both intrafollicular and intratubal overripeness, but these phenomena can also be expected to occur separately.

The frequency of affected progeny was lower when the postmenstrual period was also used for cohabitation (I A 2, I A 3 and I A 4, see fig. I). Though the numbers are very small, the ratio of pathological pregnancies to normals tends to change completely in the case of those couples who also considered the 9th and 10th day as safe (I A 5), in fact a „user failure" in a normal cycle. It is well-known that up until 1963 the first 10 days were considered safe in a cycle of 28 days. However, the ideal moment for conception is two days before the mid-cycle day (TORRANO and MURPHY 1962) and is thus closely approached, especially when the greater variability of the preovulatory phase is considered. The fact that this „user failure" leads to normal progeny is important, because there is in this case also less chance of an overripe egg, either intrafollicular or intratubal. This might even be the reason why the relation between disturbed progeny and „failure" during application of the rhythmic method did not manifest itself more clearly in the past.

Ageing of the sperm cell, while „waiting for ovulation", might also lead to pathological progeny as is shown in group I B which, although very small, is valuable since in these cases coition took place on the first day after menstruation only. Either spontaneous „early ovulations" or „provoked ovulations"

TABLE I

CATEGORY I

Applied method of rhythmic method	Number of couples	Pregnancies in spite of application of rhythmic method.							not applicable	COMPARISON GROUP: Remaining pregnancies without application of rhythmic method in the same families.						
		Normal		Pathological			Normal	Patho-logical		Normal		Pathological			Normal	Patho-logical
		Number normal children	Average maternal age at conception	Number affected children	Number abortions	Average maternal age at conception	%	%		Number normal children	Average maternal age at conception	Number affected children	Number abortions	Average maternal age at conception	%	%
Group I A																
1 coition only during premenstruum	8	1	26.7 yr.	7(6)	3	29.4 yr.	9%	91%	2	18	29.6 yr.	4(2)	7	28.3 yr.	62%	38%
2 coition after menstruation until 6th day and during premenstruum	3	1	34.6 yr.	3(3)	1	32.6 yr.	20%	80%	1	10	28.4 yr.	0	0	--	100%	0%
3 coition after menstruation until 7th day and during premenstruum	5	2	32.1 yr.	3(2)	2	29.0 yr.	29%	71%	3	13	27.11 yr.	1(1)	0	21.5 yr.	93%	7%
4 coition after menstruation until 8th day and during premenstruum	8	3	29.10 yr.	8(7)	0	32.4 yr.	27%	73%	4	18	29.3 yr.	2(0)	3	33.6 yr.	78%	22%
SUBTOTAL 1 to 4	23*	7	30.6 yr.	21(18)	6	30.5 yr.	21%	79%		55*	28.8 yr.	7(3)	9*	26.11 yr.	77%	23%
idem without propositi	23	7	--	3	6	--	44%	56%		55	--	4	9	--	81%	19%
5 coition after menstruation until 10th day and during premenstruum	6	6	30.2 yr.	1(1)	1	29.9 yr.	75%	25%	1	10	27.9 yr.	5(5)	2	28.8 yr.	41%	59%
SUBTOTAL 1 to 5	28*	13	30.4 yr.	22(19)	7	30.6 yr.	31%	69%		63*	27.8 yr.	12(8)	11	27.5 yr.	73%	27%
idem without propositi	28	13	--	3	7	--	57%	43%		63	--	4	11	--	81%	19%
Group I B coition only 1st day after menstruation	2	0	--	2(1)	0	29.6 yr.	--	--	1	2	25.4 yr.	0	1	36.2 yr.	--	--
Group I C conception just after application of rhythmic method was stopped	5	4	26.10 yr.	5(4)	1	26.10 yr.	--	--	3	5	30.2 yr.	1(1)	1	23.2 yr.	--	--
Group I D carelessly applied rhythmic method	5	1	30.0 yr.	4(4)	0	33.9 yr.	--	--	4	10	27.10 yr.	0	1	30.7 yr.	--	--
TOTAL I	35*	18	29.6 yr.	33(26)	8	30.3 yr.	31%	69%	0*	74*	30.11 yr.	12*(8*)	14*	28.7 yr.	74%	26%
idem without propositi	35	18	--	5	8	--	58%	42%	--	74	--	4	14	--	80%	20%

( ) total number of propositi; (one family with two propositi)

* The subgroups differ from each other by the varying limits of what is considered as a safe period. Some couples, for instance, after a failure went over to a more stringent form of the rhythmic method and had to be included in two different subgroups. The failure belonging to one subgroup, then, had to be scored as "not applicable" in the other. When summing the subtotals, however, couples and pregnancies were only counted once.

TABLE II

CATEGORY II

PROGENY ACCORDING TO GROUP A, B AND C. | COMPARISON GROUP: Remaining progeny in the same families.

	Number of couples	Normal — Number normal children	Normal — Average maternal age at conception	Pathological — Number affected children	Pathological — Number abortions	Pathological — Average maternal age at conception	Nor-mal %	Patho-logical %	not applicable	Normal — Number normal children	Normal — Average maternal age at conception	Pathological — Number affected children	Pathological — Number abortions	Pathological — Average maternal age at conception	Nor-mal %	Patho-logical %
A conception before return or following the first menstruation after birth or abortion	18	7	31.4 yr.	12(9)	1	29.1 yr.	35%	65%	6	76	31.6 yr.	17(11)	10	31.4 yr.	74%	26%
B born within 365 days after previous birth	10	8	30.9 yr.	5(1)	0	33.0 yr.	62%	38%	5	45	32.1 yr.	12(6)	16	35.3 yr.	62%	38%
C conception after use of oral contraceptives	2	0	--	2(1)	0	28.10 yr.	--	--	-	4	24.7 yr.	2(1)	3	27.8 yr.	--	--
TOTAL	26*	15	29.0 yr.	19(11)	1	30.1 yr.	43%	57%	1*	105*	30.8 yr.	29*(18)	23*	32.3 yr.	67%	33%
idem without propositi	26	15	--	8	1	--	62%	38%	-	105	--	11	23	--	76%	24%

CATEGORY III

PROGENY ACCORDING TO GROUP D AND E. | Remaining progeny in the same families.

	Number of couples	Normal — Number normal children	Normal — Average maternal age at conception	Pathological — Number affected children	Pathological — Number abortions	Pathological — Average maternal age at conception	Nor-mal %	Patho-logical %	not applicable	Normal — Number normal children	Normal — Average maternal age at conception	Pathological — Number affected children	Pathological — Number abortions	Pathological — Average maternal age at conception	Nor-mal %	Patho-logical %
D conception within 2 cycles after wedding date	39	20	27.3 yr.	14(11)	5	26.11 yr.	50%	50%	-	123	31.1 yr.	45(28)	27	33.8 yr.	63%	37%
idem without propositi	39	20	--	3	5	--	71%	29%	-	123	--	17	27	--	74%	26%
E premarital pregnancies	16	11	24.2 yr.	4(2)	1	23.7 yr.	69%	31%	-	46	30.0 yr.	17(14)	15	31.3 yr.	59%	41%
idem without propositi	16	11	--	2	1	--	79%	21%	-	46	--	3	15	--	72%	28%

CATEGORY IV

PROGENY ACCORDING TO GROUP F. | Remaining progeny in the same families.

	Number of couples	Normal — Number normal children	Normal — Average maternal age at conception	Pathological — Number affected children	Pathological — Number abortions	Pathological — Average maternal age at conception	Nor-mal %	Patho-logical %	not applicable	Normal — Number normal children	Normal — Average maternal age at conception	Pathological — Number affected children	Pathological — Number abortions	Pathological — Average maternal age at conception	Nor-mal %	Patho-logical %
F conception during treatment with barbiturates	5	5	27.5 yr.	6(5)	0	32.0 yr.	45%	55%	-	6	25.3 yr.	0	1	26.8 yr.	86%	14%
idem without propositi	5	5	--	1	0	--	83%	17%	-	6	--	0	1	--	86%	14%

CATEGORY V

The frequency of intercourse was indicated as very low (± < 1 per cycle):

- due to the illness or absence of one of the partners : 2 propositi and 1 abortion
- by very sporadic premarital contacts : 2 propositi
- in elderly couples : 4 propositi

Failure during the application of coitus interruptus : 5 propositi
Failure during the application of coitus condomatus : 2 propositi and 1 abortion

( ) total number of propositi

* As some couples were included in both groups A, B and C a correction had to be made for the total.

caused by copulation should be postulated here (Bickenbach et al. 1960).

As far as group I C is concerned, one should also consider the possibility of premenstrual conception, since in 2 out of 5 pathological cases birth occurred 4 weeks earlier than calculated and the birth weight was in disproportion with the supposedly shortened duration of gestation. In addition, Marshall (1968) points out the tendency of parents to justify a pregnancy occurring while applying the rhythmic method, by stating that this pregnancy was in fact wanted. Together with group I D these could be grouped as „accidental pregnancies". Here, too, we observe a rise in congenital deviations.

In conclusion, it is seen that 35 couples, while practising the rhythmic method as a means of contraception, had no less than 59 pregnancies, of which 69 % resulted in an abnormal outcome.

If the „user failures" (I A 5) and the „accidental pregnancies" (I C and I D) are excluded, the number of „biological failures" (I A 1, I A 2, I A 3, I A 4 and I B) is approached and the trend becomes increasingly clear: 81 % „pathological" and 19 % „normal." In the 74 remaining pregnancies in the same families, conceived without application of the rhythmic method, the ratio was totally reversed: 77 % „normal" and 23 % „pathological". These figures have a limited reliability due to the fact that this is a retrospective investigation in which the parents might twist the issue. This, however, is compensated for by the clear differences with the „comparison" groups in the same families.

From the average age of the mother at conception (see table I) it is seen that pathological progeny caused by biological failures during practice of the rhythmic method is not age-dependent. There is no clear difference between this average and the average for this country as can be seen from data from the Central Bureau for Statistics: from 1961 until 1966 (without 1963) the average maternal age at delivery was 29 years for all births together. It should be noted here that in our tables abortions were also included when calculating the average age of the mother at conception. In addition we must take into account that at a more advanced age contraception is applied more frequently and more strictly than before, as by this stage the family is usually already formed.

That pathological pregnancies, occurring in spite of application of the rhythmic method, are probably due to fertilization of an intrafollicularly aged egg, can be seen from fig. I. It is evident that the frequency of pathological progeny was highest when copulation only took place during the premenstrual period, and that it falls the more the preovulatory phase is used. The following anamnestic data also suggest the fertilization of an egg ovulating late in the cycle: vomiting during the „last menstruation", movements of the child at „3½ months" and „premature" birth of a too heavy baby. All this

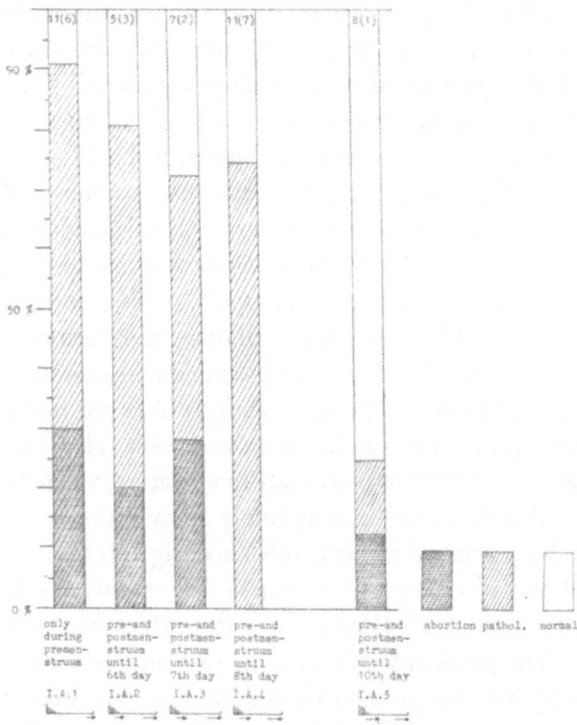

Fig. 1. The abnormal progeny decreases when the „safe period" is extended into the postmenstrual phase. At the top of the graph the number of pregnancies, and between brackets the number of propositi are indicated.

can be explained using IFFY's (1962, 1963 and 1968) hypothesis of late post-ovulatory conception. In such cases the next menstruation could no longer be suppressed so that the woman, ignorant of the already existing pregnancy, made a wrong calculation concerning the expected birthdate.

LANMAN (1968) voiced, on the basis of animal experiments collected from the literature, the opinion that the rhythmic method in man should lead to congenital malformations, although no cases were known to him. In the extensive literature on the application of the rhythmic method little attention has been paid to the consequences for the progeny of „failure" in the method (HARTMAN 1962, DÖRING 1967 and MARSHALL 1968). Only BARTZEN (1967) analyses these pregnancy products, separating „teaching errors", „calculated risks" and „system failures". His first group (32 pregnancies) could correspond somewhat with the group described by us as I A 5 (user failures). His second group of „calculated risks" (41 pregnancies) is not relevant as we have to do with a retrospective investigation. The „system failures", however, analogous with

31

the „biological failures" reported here, receive little attention. The smallness of this group in BARTZEN's paper (6 pregnancies on 4.824 cycles) is sharply contrasted with the great number of „biological failures" found in this investigation. This does suggest that the progeny resulting from such a „failure" is concentrated in institutes for mental defectives. It should be noted also that in BARTZEN's investigation the parents concerned combined the rhythmic method with basal body temperature control, which undoubtedly decreases the chance of „biological failures". In the 35 couples interrogated by us only 2 used this control at the time of conception. An analysis of these temperature lists was no longer possible as they had been destroyed. KOHANE's et al. (1967) comment concerning the dissociation of increased temperature and ovulation fits in here too. Using culdoscopy these authors observed that in some cases after a temperature rise no corpus luteum was present. They concluded from this that the data obtained from basal body temperature, vaginal cytology and cervical arborization do not necessarily imply an ovulation.

It has already been assumed by many other investigators that a great variation in the postovulatory phase is possible, even in the successive cycles of a „regularly menstruating woman" (HARTMAN 1962, MARSHALL 1963, BELL and LORAINE 1965). The possibility of premenstrual conception has been emphasized especially by IFFY. According to him these „post-mid-cycle conceptions" have at times resulted in pathological pregnancies, such as tubal pregnancy, mola hydatidosa and abortion (1962, 1963 and 1968). Moreover, it has been known for a long time that ripe Graafian follicles can be present at the end of the cycle and that conceptions can also take place in that period. STIEVE (1950) mentioned the possibility of ovulation after the mid-cycle and called this phenomenon „paracyclic ovulation", while REIMANN-HUNZIGER and WILD pointed to various cases of „secondary ovulation" (1963).

II. Special attention should be paid to the pregnancies occurring before or after the first menstruation following birth or abortion (II A), of which 65 % were pathological: one abortion and 12 congenital anomalies, including 9 propositi. To approach the problem as correctly as possible we collected in addition in II B all the births that took place within a year after the previous birth or abortion without the parents being able to remember the number of menstruations that had occurred between the pregnancies concerned. Thus we are mainly dealing here with pregnancies resulting from the fertilization of either the first or the second ovulation. The percentage of pathological pregnancies in this group, although high, is not higher than it is in the „comparison group" with all other pregnancies in the same families, where the birth interval was longer than one year. It should also be pointed out that the figures in II B are levelled to some extent by the fact that some couples with a great number of conceptions could not remember the exact time interval between birth or lactation and the following abortion. Consequently, we could not include in this group those cases of abortion that had only been suspected. By adding II A to II B the higher frequency of pathological pregnancies remains clear: 55 % versus 32 % of all the remaining pregnancies in the same families. Finally, we should like to draw attention to the 2 pathological pregnancies occurring after the use of ovulation inhibitors (II C). In this category, too, there was no clear dependency on the mothers' age.

It is generally found that the first ovulation after a birth with or without lactation (LYON and STAMM 1946, CHARTIER and GILLAIN 1964, SALBER et al. 1966 and SHARMAN 1966), after an abortion (SHARMAN 1966) or after the use of ovulation inhibitors (SHEARMAN 1964, RICE-WRAY et al. 1967 and MEARS 1968) usually starts only hesitantly. The follicular phase is then often protracted and the luteal phase shortened by a corpus luteum insufficiency. In all these situations some cycles can pass without ovulation, and even extended periods of secondary amenorrhea are known. The latter can be treated with gonadotrophines or clomiphen (SHEARMAN 1964, 1966 and 1968). Investigation concerning lactation in under-developed countries, where long periods of infertility are encountered especially in the lower strata of the population, have shown that nutrition plays an important role. Analogous data were obtained for rabbits (ADAMS 1967) and beef-cows (OXENREIDER 1968) where treatment with gonadotrophines can also start off the ovulation. The situation in man during lactation is in fact even more complex, as is shown by the fact that a normal FSH and LH rhythm can be restored without an actual ovulation taking place (KELLER 1968). This might indicate that during lactation the target organs of the hypothalamus-pituitary-ovary axis are less sensitive or even refractory to the normal physiological stimulus of the gonadotrophines. Consequently, the egg cell is in a precarious position in the first, and possibly the second, ovulation. After a period of suppression the coördinated hypothalamic and pituitary functions have to start working again to restore the very complicated hormonal balance and the clockwork mechanism of the FSH-oestrogen and LH-progesteron cycle. As a second step the ovaries have to escape from their compulsory refractoriness to resume optimal functioning. These complicated phenomena could prolong the ripening of the first (and following) egg, thus increasing the chance of overripeness.

In this connection it is important to mention that MORICARD (1967), while looking for the correct proportion of FSH and LH necessary to provoke ovulation in infant mice, concluded that these gonadotrophines have to be administered in quantitatively and chronologically very narrowly limited proportions

Over and above he repeatedly observed normal and abnormal ovocytes, the latter partially segmented after provocation of an ovulation. In man also a rise is seen in abortions and multiple pregnancies after provocation of ovulation, both with gonadotrophines (RABAU et al. 1967, 1969) and clomiphen (JOHNSON et al. 1966). Studies of these data show that out of 301 pregnancies arising in the first month after clomiphen treatment, 35 multiple pregnancies (8.6 %) and 122 abortions, together with premature births (40 %), occurred. A month later these deviations dropped to respectively 0.7 % and 23 %, which is within normal limits. About the children themselves no data are given, except that „no rise in congenital deviations was found". It should be remembered, however, that e.g. congenital deviations of the central nervous system can remain latent during the first months and even years of life. There has been no follow-up study on these children.

Literature concerning ovulation during the puerperal period pays no attention to the resulting fertilization of the egg concerned. Some cases of misformed progeny with notation of the time interval since the previous birth are cited by DEKIGAI et al. (1968) and FUJIMOTO (1968). Furthermore, different authors (ROCHESTER 1923, YERUSHALMY 1945 and 1956) showed that the perinatal mortality rate was higher when the interval between births was short. EASTMAN (1944) was able to demonstrate a relatively high rate when the interval between births was under 12 months, but found no increase in the rate for other intervals. JAMES (1968) therefore uses the data collected in „the Perinatal Mortality Survey" and tabulated the pregnancies against the interval between these confinements and the preceding ones: 6 to 12 months, 13 to 18 months, 19 to 24 months etc. From these data it is possible to calculate the ratio of the „perinatal mortality" of all pregnancies in each of the above interval-groups. This shows that in the interval within the year (6 to 12) this is 49 %, while it drops in the following groups to 25 % (13 to 18 months) and 23 % (18 to 24 months). In other words, the pregnancies occurring during the first cycles after the previous partus carry a far greater risk. The author analyses these data but attempts to minimise their significance by calling them the result of statistical artifacts, although he does admit that attempts to explain these findings should certainly be justified. We feel that the overripeness theory fits in well here.

CARR (1967 and 1969) and BOUÉ (1968) mention chromosomal aberrations in abortions of women becoming pregnant after use of ovulation inhibitors. Other authors include multiple and ectopic pregnancies and in addition malformed progeny in this framework (HETHERINGTON 1947 and THOMPSON 1969). In reviews on pregnancies occurring after the use of ovulation inhibitors the relation to aberrant progeny has hardly been investigated (WATTS et al. 1964,

RICE-WRAY et al. 1965 and 1966, SURAN 1967 and GARCIA 1968). To our knowledge no follow-up studies have been carried out on these „viable children without gross congenital abnormalities". In this connection we would like to draw attention to one of our patients who was conceived in the first month after stopping with the use of an oral ovulation inhibitor (Anovlar ®). The patient in question is an aphatic, imbecile boy of 5 years without any gross congenital malformation, but suffering from epilepsy and clear neurological damages in the region of the cranial nerves. In our experience these small congenital aberrations of the cerebral nervous system tend to be recognized only when the child becomes older. A second remark we wish to make is that in the reviews the time interval between termination of the use of oral contraceptives and the beginning of pregnancy is often ignored. It is necessary to pay attention to this factor, since there might be shown to exist a negative correlation between the number of abnormal pregnancies and the rise in the number of cycles after withdrawal of the contraceptive drug.

III. It has been shown repeatedly in many investigations into the connection between birth number and frequency of abortions, still-births, congenital deviations and mental retardation, that first pregnancies are a heavily taxed group, for which there is yet no satisfactory explanation. Among our 127 couples there were 39 in which a pregnancy occurred within the first two months after marriage. Of these 50 % were pathological. This is an indication that the wellknown risk of primiparity is mainly confined to a limited period just after marriage. This became increasingly clear when it was investigated in which month after the marriage conception took place, Naturally, couples having had premarital intercourse had to be excluded. Consequently, 101 couples remained, out of whom 63 women conceived during the first four months. The ratio of pathological to healthy progeny expressed in percentages is shown in fig. 2. The progressive drop after the first month is striking.

This phenomenon might possibly be explained by intratubal overripeness after the ovulation during the first cycle, which doubtlessly must arise because the first coition can take place in the days following the ovulation. An additional factor, more important in our view, is „stress". We have already mentioned that several women remembered that they had menstruated on their wedding day against their expectations. The fact that „stress" has a disregulating effect on the cycle and ovulation is well known to the layman, but has only recently been critically investigated (KOHANE 1967 and DALTON 1968). We mentioned previously that a disturbance of the cycle can also influence the following cycle (DÖRING 1967).

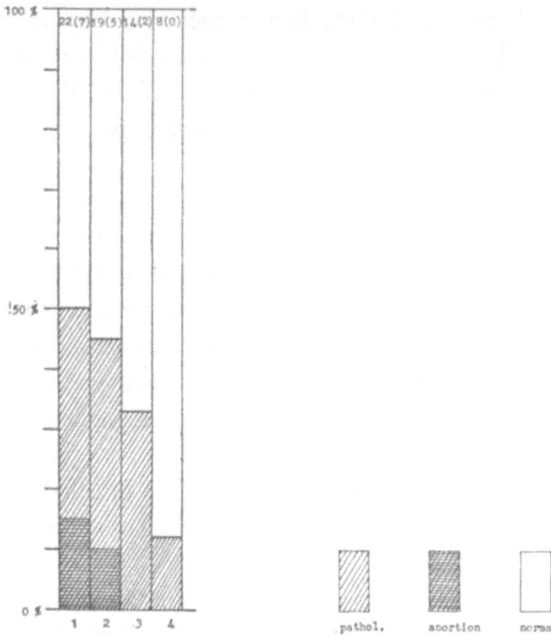

Fig. 2. The month of conception of the first pregnancy in 63 couples, having had no prenuptial contact is set out horizontally (see text). The conception fell within the first four months of marriage, respectively 22, 19, 14 and 8 times. At the top of the graph the number of propositi is indicated between brackets. The percentage of pathological and normal progeny is compared. The progressive drop after the first month of marriage is striking.

IV. In the very small group of 5 couples in which the mother was treated with barbiturates for epilepsy or nervousness, the occurrence of pathological pregnancies was striking, especially when compared with pregnancies from the period when they were not treated with these drugs (see comparison group in table II: 55 % versus 14 %). Although the trend shown in this table could be explained by an age-dependent effect, we do not believe that this was the case. Two of the mothers concerned had already produced normal offspring before treatment became necessary. The figures are too small, however, to allow definite conclusions to be drawn. Nevertheless, this group becomes significant in the light of the problem posed by MEADOW (1968) concerning children born to mothers treated with anti-epileptica. He did not suspect barbiturates then, but primidone as teratogenic during the pregnancy and not before pregnancy. BIRD (1969), however, stated that he had never observed congenital deviations in children of mothers treated with antiepileptic drugs.

Against this statement the same objection can be raised as previously, since, in order to be absolutely certain, a follow-up study of at least 5 years' duration would be necessary, as congenital deviations of e.g. the central nervous system are often overlooked in the first years of life.

Why then this suspicion of barbiturates? EVERETT and SAWYER (1950) discovered a method which, via the hypothalamus, prevented or delayed ovulation and luteinisation of the follicle in the rat. These methods were used later, by FUGO and BUTCHER (1966, 1967 and 1969) in their experiments concerning intrafollicular overripeness of the egg, in which they observed a clear rise of the number of abnormally developing zygotes with or without chromosomal deviations. To do this they administered parenterally a daily dose of phenobarbital of 50 mg. per kg. An equivalent dose applied to an adult human being would be exceptionally high, namely 3 g. per day. This, however, does not offer sufficient information about the dosage in man, so that the action of a low dosage over longer periods needs further study. EVERETT and SAWYER (1955) also prevented ovulation by means of other compounds, such as anticholinergics, antiadrenergics and also morphine, pharmaceuticals with varying actions but probably exerting in this respect a similar influence via the reticular system.

Animal experiments have shown that neuroleptics as well have a point of attack in the hypothalamic-pituitary-gonadal system. Reserpine and chloropromazines can retard FSH and LH hormones and at the same time stimulate the production of prolactine, which is also produced by the frontal lobe of the pituitary gland. DE WIED (1967), reviewing animal experiments, notes after the administration of neuroleptics to the mother animal an elaborate spectrum of defective reproduction: infertility, abortion, increased intrauterine death and still-births. In man, too, disregulation of the menstrual cycle after the use of neuroleptics is well-known, in fact a daily experience in psychiatric units (PY and MATHIEU 1960 and PLANTE and ROY 1967). WHITELAW (1956) could, with a dose of chlorpromazine (25 mg. twice daily), delay the menstruation of women with a regular cycle by 8 to 16 days. This phenomenon could only be elicited when the dose was administered 1 to 3 days before the expected ovulation.

Returning to our cases we should point out that 2 of the 4 propositi were conceived in spite of the application of the rhythmic method. In both these cases the administration of barbiturates might perhaps have been the cause of the „biological failure", by delaying ovulation and enabling fertilization at a later moment.

V. The last group is the most speculative, but not without importance. The connection between decreased coition frequency and defective progeny was suggested by HARTMAN (1962) and, as far as Down's syndrome is concerned, by GERMAN (1968). In the mammal the sperm is present in the area of the ovaries when the ripe egg cell is released, so that it can then be fertilized. Decrease in coition frequency in man, especially around ovulation time, does suggest theoretically that the egg could become overripe in the tube before being fertilized. This could be one facet of the increased frequency of abortions, still-births and congenital deviations in older couples, where coition frequency has usually decreased. Another facet is the increased chance of intra-follicular overripeness, since in many premenopausal women the cycle becomes irregular and even anovulatory, because of a disturbance in the functioning of the hypothalamic-pituitary-gonadal system.

In the case of decreased coition frequency the possibility of intratubal ageing of the sperm must also be included, as has been pointed out earlier. It is also important to realize that in pregnancies occurring in spite of coitus interruptus and any other form of contraception, similar complications as in the case of decreased coition frequency could play a part.

It is evident that besides the factors responsible for pathological progeny in the well-known high risk group of the elderly woman, there are others which are age-independent. A bimodal age distribution of these two components has been shown to exist for trisomy 18 (HECHT et al. 1963 and TAYLOR 1967), for Down's syndrome (PENROSE 1966) and for trisomy D_1 (MAGENIS et al. 1968). The first component of such a curve conforms with the distribution of maternal age in the general population. The second is a reflection of the age-dependent factors that play a role in the origin of such progeny. Consequently, to explain these observations, age-independent as wel as age-dependent mechanisms were suggested, both, however, leading to the same result. The over-ripeness theory might offer an explanation for the bimodality of the age distribution curve, since overripeness of the egg and intratubal ageing of the sperm can occur in young married couples. These phenomena might even be induced under various conditions, as we attempted to show in our investigation. The „high risks" concerned might also occur in the second peak of the bimodal curve along with the increased lability of the premenopausal menstrual cycle and the decrease in coition frequency, factors which may normally be expected in this age group.

In the 127 couples studied we observed the following age-independent and, in our opinion, up till now unknown „high risk" groups:

1. biological failures during the rhythmic method;
2. pregnancies conceived immediately post abortum, post partum or during nursing and after use of hormonal steroids;
3. pregnancies within two cycles after marriage.

In addition we pointed out that on the basis of our investigation and the data in the literature the chances to have defective progeny might possibly be higher in mothers using barbiturates and neuroleptics before conception. Sporadic sexual intercourse was also mentioned as a possibility. Reduced coition frequency, due to temporary absence or illness of one of the partners or to the increase of the number of years of marriage, might also cause an increase in defective progeny. Another wellknown high-risk group is the progeny of mothers with hypothyroidism, caused among others by autoimmune disease of the thyroid gland (Hashimoto's disease) (FIALKOW et al. 1965 and DALLAIRE et al. 1969). It is known that in hypothyroidism more cases of amenorrhea, menorrhagia and also of sterility occur. Both histological and biological investigations have shown that in these cases there exists a corpus luteum deficiency which can be remedied by the administration of thyroid extracts. An ovopathy, due to disregulation of the hypothalamus-pituitary-ovary axis, might well be the cause of the increased risk of defective progeny.

This train of thought could also be useful in explaining the rise in the number of congenital malformations from diabetic mothers. Symptomatic hypoglycemia in itself does not seem to lead to malformations (FARQUHAR 1969). One might, however, expect a disturbance in the ovulation pattern of diabetics and prediabetics on the basis of the interrelations between glucocorticoids and ovulation (JEFFERIES 1966).

It is not impossible that a rise in the frequency of mongolism nine months after an epidemic of viral hepatitis could be due to a disturbance in the ovulation, leading to ovopathy. Recurrent abortions also have to be considered, since they are often linked with a prevalence of congenital aberrations. The data of DALLA PRIA et al. (1967) point in the same direction, as they found in the majority of women having recurrent abortions a corpus luteum deficiency, and disturbances in the oestrogens.

A most interesting point is that all high-risk groups can be brought under a common denominator, viz. firstly a disturbance in ovulation, in other words an increased chance of intrafollicular overripeness, and secondly, a disturbance in time of fertilization, in other words an increased chance of intratubal overripeness.

In the group of mentally retarded patients reported here the enquiry after moment and circumstances of fertilization suggested in about half of the cases an overripe egg. Consequently, we postulate that this phenomenon is a very important cause of mental retardation. Therefore, in an institution for the mentally retarded one can expect to find the results of „conceptopathology" in the normal population. Several investigations into the prevalence of conceptopathology in normal populations are under way.

A tentative approach to this prevalence in the normal population might be obtained from the percentages calculated without propositi (tables I and II). This preliminary estimate is, as mentioned above, certainly too high, especially in the first category, since having a retarded child, whatever the aetiology, will strongly influence the parents both in their motives for family planning and in the strictness of the method used. The application of the rhythmic method, as stated, might increase the chances of fertilization of an overripe egg and intratubal ageing of sperm. Furthermore, one should also take into account the constitution of certain women, namely the lability of the complex endocrinological system that regulates the ovulation. These two factors lead us to expect a greater prevalence of „conceptopathology" in our group, compared with the normal population.

As far as the nature of the aberrations in the patients with a „positive overripeness–anamnesis" is concerned, there is a great variety. Both numerical and structural deviations of the chromosomes have been found, as well as cases without chromosomal deviations. It seems that overripeness of the egg cell can have teratogenic as well as mutagenic consequences. We found patients with respectively congenital hypothyroidism, atypical (sporadically occurring) ectodermal dysplasia, Hallermann-Streiff's syndrome, Silver's syndrome, Prader-Willi's syndrome, Goldenhar's syndrome twice, „male Turner" syndrome, meningomyelocele and further clino-, micro- and dyscephalias and many other malformations hard to define. The anamnesis convinced us every time that ovopathy was a possibility, especially in all those cases where the aetiology has not yet been explained. The study of the clinical syndromes and their gradual transitions is very stimulating. In addition we found the „overripeness–anamnesis" positive in eight children with Down's syndrome and in patients with respectively an acentric extra chromosome, a ring-G chromosome, a deletion in chromosome 4, a deletion in chromosome 5 and a structural aberration in an X- or a C-group chromosome. A great number of our propositi were registered as victims of pregnancy pathology and neonatal disturbances, while the conception anamnesis led us to a deeper insight. No indications, however, were found of positive „overripeness–anamnesis" in the seven cases of postnatal encephalitis and the two cases of perinatal hyperbilirubinemia.

We may conclude that, although in man the teratogenic and mutagenic action of overripeness of the egg cell has not been proved, there are sufficiently strong indications to accept it as a hypothesis. This can be a very useful approach to the causes of abortion, still-births, congenital deviations, multiple births and psychomotoric retardation with or without chromosomal deviations. It is also to be expected that psychopathology of unknown origin and many „minor defects" can arise in this way. The viewpoints stated here are not facts established above all doubt, as there are still so many uncertainties, but it is hoped that further research will solve these in time. If the results of these investigations are confirmed in principle by others, then certain socio-hygienic measures could be formulated with important consequences for the prophylaxis in human progeny. It is also to be expected that such results will influence the interpretation of human genetical problems.

I should like to thank the medical students Miss M. Arends, Y. Margry and M. Strankinga and Mr. H. Homans for their coöperation in checking the material and their help in drawing up this article. Prof. Dr. T. D. Stahlie, Prof. Dr. G. Godefroy and Dr. E. G. Bijnen, statistician, are thanked for their critical remarks. Thanks are also due to Mr. G. van der Most, medical director of the institute „Huize Maria Roepaan" for stimulating this work, and to my colleagues C. van Kempen, J. Lormans and J. Maas who enabled me to compile these results. Mrs. S. Lormans, Dr. C. van Kempen and Mr. G. Hamers are thanked for their metabolic and cytogenetical investigations, Mrs. G. A. van der Meij, B. Sc., for the translation into English and Mrs. E. Lely-van Baal for drawing the diagrams.

SUMMARY

To test the hypotheses formulated earlier concerning the overripeness of the egg we questioned 127 couples with one or more mentally retarded children to enquire after the time and circumstances under which conception took place. Attention was paid to all pregnancies, whether or not resulting in an abortion, a mentally retarded or a normal child.

A clear correlation was seen between the occurrence of pathological progeny and „biological failures" during the application of the rhythmic method without basal body temperature control. Furthermore the same correlations were seen to exist in conceptions occurring immediately post abortum, post partum or durante lactatione. Attention was also paid to conceptions occurring immediately after use of ovulation inhibitors and during treatment with barbiturates. It is generally well-known that primiparous mothers run a greater risk to produce abnormal progeny. This risk was seen to be increased for pregnancies which originated in the first or second cycle after marriage. In the above mentioned situations, where on theoretical grounds overripeness of the ovocyte could be expected, a definite increase in pathological progeny has been established. Therefore we became more and more convinced that this pathological progeny could only be understood by assuming that in these situations the chances of a deterioration of the egg are increased, due especially to pre- and/or postovulatory overripeness. The already known „high risk categories" such as mothers with diabetes, with thyroid abnormalities or of increased age, and all conceptions during virus epidemics (hepatitis), might be brought under the same heading.

These observations, made in a population from an institute for mental defectives, may show the results of „conceptopathology" probably occurring in normal society.

The consequences of these new studies on certain aspects of mental retardation are particularly interesting. They throw a new light both on the origin of a great number of types of mental retardation, which were up till now aetiologically hard to understand, and possibly also on some forms of human psychopathology. Furthermore, not only the teratogenic, but also the mutagenic action is emphasized through which chromosomal aberrations can arise, including reciprocal translocations which can be inherited for several generations.

If these results could be confirmed, then this could lead to a number of prophylactic measures of great importance for public health, thereby exerting a definite influence on human genetic problems.

SAMENVATTING

Teneinde de hypothesen, die vroeger werden geformuleerd aangaande de overrijpheid van de eicel, te toetsen, hebben wij 127 echtparen met één of meer mentaal geretardeerde kinderen ondervraagd ter informatie omtrent het tijdstip waarop, en de omstandigheden waarin de conceptie plaats vond. Daarbij werd aandacht besteed aan al hun zwangerschappen, ongeacht of het om een abortus, een gestoord of een normaal kind ging.

Wij zagen bij de pathologische progenituur een duidelijke correlatie met „biological failures" tijdens toepassing van periodieke onthouding zonder basale lichaamstemperatuurcontrole. Verder werden dezelfde correlaties geconstateerd met concepties post abortum, post partum sive durante lactatione. Aandacht werd ook besteed aan de concepties onmiddellijk na gebruik van ovulatieremmers en tijdens behandeling met barbituraten. Dat eerstbarenden een groter risico lopen op abnormale progenituur is algemeen bekend. Het bleek dat dit risico het grootst was bij zwangerschappen die in de eerste of tweede cyclus na de huwelijkssluiting tot stand kwamen. In al de beschreven situaties, waarin op theoretische gronden overrijping van de eicel kan worden verwacht, werd dus een stijging van pathologische progenituur vastgesteld. Daarom groeide onze overtuiging dat deze pathologische progenituur alleen kan worden begrepen doordat in de bedoelde situaties de kansen op vermindering van kwaliteit van de eicel zijn gestegen, met name door preovulatoire of/en post-ovulatoire overrijpheid. Ook reeds eerder bekende „high risks" bij moeders met diabetes of met schildklierafwijkingen, bij moeders op gevorderde leeftijd en verder ook concepties tijdens virale hepatitisepidemieën, kunnen onder dezelfde noemer worden gebracht.

Deze bevindingen in een populatie binnen een instituut voor zwakzinnigen, laten zien dat deze instituten een concentratie bevatten van de gevolgen van wat zich aan conceptiepathologie in de normale samenleving afspeelt.

De consequenties van deze nieuwe bestuderingswijze van de symptomatologie bij psychomotorisch geretardeerde patiënten zijn buitengewoon interessant. Zij werpen een nieuw licht op de ontstaanswijze van een groot aantal tot nu toe etiologisch ondoorzichtige zwakzinnigheidsbeelden en wellicht ook van sommige vormen van menselijke psychopathologie. Niet alleen wordt op de teratogene, maar ook op de mutagene werking gewezen, waardoor chromosomenafwijkingen kunnen ontstaan, inbegrepen reciproke translokaties die in verschillende generaties kunnen worden overgeërfd.

Indien deze resultaten door anderen worden bevestigd, kan dit leiden tot een aantal profylactische maatregelen, die van groot belang kunnen zijn voor de volksgezondheid. Ook het genetisch denken kan hierdoor beïnvloed worden.

LITERATURE

ADAMS, C. E., Concurrent lactation and pregnancy in the rabbit. *J. Reprod. Fertil.* 14: 351, 1967.
BARTZEN, P. J., Effectiveness of the Temperature Rhythm-system of contraception. *Fertil. Steril.* 18: 694, 1967.
BELL, E. T. and J. A. LORAINE, Time of ovulation in relation to cycle length. *Lancet*, 1: 1029, 1965.
BICKENBACH, W., G. K. DÖRING and C. HOSSFELD, Experimentelle Frühovulation durch Cervixreizung beim Menschen. *Archiv für Gynäkol.* 192: 412, 1960.
BIRD, A. V., Anticonvulsant drugs and congenital abnormalities. *Lancet*, i: 311, 1969.
BOUE, J. G., J. COHEN, J. HENRY-SUCHET, R. MERGER and C. VINCENT, Etude clinique et biologique de 16 cas d'avortements spontanés par aberration chromosomique. *La presse médicale*, 76: 1717, 1968.
BUTCHER, R. L., and N. W. FUGO, Overripeness and the Mammalian Ova II. Delayed ovulation and chromosome anomalies. *Fertil. Steril* 18: 297, 1967.

BUTCHER, R. L., J. D. BLUE and N. W. FUGO, III. Fetal development at midgestation and at term. *Fertil. Steril.* 20: 223, 1969.

CARR, D. H., Chromosomes after oral contraceptives. *Lancet*, ii: 830, 1967.

CARR D. H., *Chromosomal abnormalities in clinical medicine, Progress in Medical Genetics*. Ed. A. G. Steinberg & A. G. Bearn. IV: 1, 1969, New York and Londen.

CHARTIER, M. and M. GILLAIN, Post-partum et courbe thermique à propos de 281 observations. *Bull. Soc. Roy. Belge Gynec.* 34: 271, 1964.

CRONIN, T. J., Influence of lactation upon ovulation. *Lancet*, ii: 422, 1968.

DALLAIRE, L., D. KINGSMILL-FLYNN and G. LEBOEUF, Autoimmunity and chromosomal aberrations. *Can. Med. J. Ass.* 100: 1, 1969.

DALLA PRIA, S., D. MINUCCI and G. PELUSI, L'incidensa dell' ipoluteinismo e del ciclo anovulatorio in un gruppo di donne soggette ad aborto abituale indagine colpocitologica. *Riv. Ital. Ginec.* 51: 470, 1967.

DALTON, K., Menstruation and examination. *Lancet*, ii: 1386, 1968.

DEKIGAI, K., S. U. WANG, F. OKANO, Incidence of spina bifida in three consecutive babies. *Advances Obstet. Gynec.* 20: 311, 1968.

DÖRING, G. K., Uber die Zuverlässigkeit der Temperaturmethode zur Empfängnisverhütung. *Dtsch. med. Wschr.* 92: 1056, 1967.

EASTMAN, N. J., The effect of the interval between births on maternal and fetal outlook. *Am. J. Obst. Gynec.* 47: 445, 1944.

EVERETT, J. W. and CH. H. SAWYER, A 24-hour periodicity in the „L.H.-release apparatus" of female rats, disclosed by barbiturate sedation. *Endocrinol.* 47: 198, 1950.

FARQUHAR, J. W., Prognosis for babies born to diabetic mothers in Edinburgh. *Arch. Dis. Childh.*, 44: 36, 1969.

FIALKOW, P. J., I. UCHIDA, F. HECHT en A. G. MOTULSKY, Increased frequency of thyreoid antibodies in mothers of patients with Down's syndrome. *Lancet*, ii: 868, 1965.

FUGO, N. W. and R. L. BUTCHER, Overripeness and the mammalian ova. I. Overripeness and early embryonic development. *Fertil. Steril.* 17: 804, 1966.

FUJIMOTO, A., A case of syrenomelus. *Advances Obstet. Gynec.* 20: 307, 1968.

GARCIA, C. R. and A. DAVID, Long-term effects of oral contraceptives on the ovary and pituitary. *Fertil. Steril.* 13: 287, 1968.

GERMAN, J., Mongolism, delayed fertilization and human sexual behavior. *Nature* 217: 516, 1968.

HARTMAN, C. G., *Science and the safe period*. The Williams and Wilkins Company, Baltimore, 1962.

HECHT, F., J. S. BRYANT, A. G. MOTULSKY and E. R. GIBLETT, The No. 17—18 (E) trisomy syndrome. *J. Pediat.* 63: 605, 1963.

HETHERINGTON, R. J., Chromosomes after oral contraception. *Lancet*, ii: 897, 1967.

IFFY, L. and P. KERNER, The aetiology of early abortion. *J. Obst. Gynaec. Brit. Commonw.* 69: 598, 1962.

IFFY, L., The time of conception in pathological gestations. *Proc. Roy. Soc. Med.* 56: 1098, 1963.

IFFY, L., Recent investigation concerning the aetiology of ectopic pregnancies. *Aust. N. Z. J. Obstet. Gynaec.* 8: 131, 1968.

JAMES, W. H., Stillbirth, neonatal death and birth interval. *Ann. Hum. Genet. Lond.* 32: 163, 1968.

JEFFERIES, W. MCK., *Glucocorticoids and ovulation. Ovulation*, p. 62. Ed. M. B. Greenblatt, J. B. Lippincott company, 1966.

JOHNSON, J. E. JR., C. A. BUNDE and M. T. HOEKENGA, Clinical experience with clomiphene. *Pacif. med. and Surg.* 74: 153, 1966.

JONGBLOET, P. H., Overripeness of the egg. *Maandschr. Kindergeneesk.* 36: 352, 1968.

JONGBLOET, P. H., Overrijpheid van het ovum. *Ned. T. Geneesk.* 113: 653, 1969. *Ibidem* 113: 1215, 1969.

KELLER, P. J., Excretion of F.S.H. and L.H. during lactation. *Acta Endocr.* 57: 529, 1968.

LANMAN, J. T., Delays during reproduction and their effects on the embryo and fetus. 2. Aging of Eggs. *N. Engl. J. Med.* 278: 1047, 1968.

LEADING article, Human gonadotrophins in the treatment of infertility. *Lancet* i: 1182, 1969.

KOHANE, E. S., M. SHARF and T. KUZMINSKY, The use of H.C.G. in delayed ovulation during artificial insemination. *Fertil. Steril.* 18: 593, 1967.

LYON, R. A. and M. J. STAMM, The onset of ovulation during the puerperium. *Calif. Med.* 65: 99, 1946.

MAGENIS, R. E., F. HECHT and S. MILHAM, Trisomy 13 (D$_1$) Syndrome: Studies on parental age, sex ratio, and survival. *J. Pediat.* 73: 222, 1968.

MARSHALL, J., Thermal changes in the normal menstrual cycle. *Brit. Med. J.* I: 102, 1963.

MARSHALL, J., A field trial of the basal-body-temperature method of regulating births. *Lancet,* ii: 8, 1968.

MEADOW, S. R., Anticonvulsant drugs and congenital abnormalities. *Lancet,* ii: 1296, 1968.

MEARS, E., Pregnancy following antifertility agents. *Intern. J. of Fertil.* 13: 340, 1968.

MIKAMO, K., Intrafollicular overripeness and teratologic development. *Cytogenetics* 7: 212, 1968.

MORICARD, R., Gonadotrophines, méiose et ovulation. Cytophysiologie et applications humaines. *Rev. franç. Gynéc.* 62: 591, 1967.

OXENREIDER, S. L., Effects of suckling and ovarian function on postpartum reproductive activity in beef cows. *Am. J. Vet. Res.* 29: 2099, 1968.

PENROSE, L. S. and G. F. SMITH, *Down's anomaly,* Boston, 1966, Little, Brown & Company.

PLANTE, N. and P. ROY, Galactorrhée et neuroleptiques. *Laval méd.* 38: 103, 1967.

PY, O. and P. MATHIEU, Galactorrhée et troubles du cycle menstruel au cours de traitements neuroleptiques. *La presse médicale* 68: 765, 1960.

RABAU, E., A. DAVID, D. M. SERR, S. MASHIACH and B. LUNENFELD, Human menopausal gonadotropins for anovulation and sterility. *Am. J. Obst. Gynec.* 98: 92, 1967.

REIMANN-HUNZIGER, R. and W. WILD, Indicine-Hormonal birth control on a natural basis. *J. Reprod. Fertil.* 6: 175, 1963.

RICE-WRAY, E., Fertility after use of oral antifertility agents and health of children born to these mothers. Research on steroids, ed. by C. Cassano, p. 525. *Il Pensiero Scientifico,* Roma, 1966.

RICE-WRAY, E., S. CORREU, J. GORODOVSKY, J. ESQUIVEL and. J. W. GOLDZIEHER, Return of ovulation after discontinuance of oral contraceptives. *Fertil. Steril.* 18: 212, 1967.

ROCHESTER, A., *Infant Mortality.* Publication no. 119 of the Children's Bureau, U.S. Dept. of Labor, Washington, 1923.

SALBER, E. J., M. FEINLEIB and B. MACMAHON, The duration of postpartum amenorrhea. *Am. J. Epidem.* 82: 347, 1965.

SAWYER, CH. H., B. V. CRITCHILOW and CH. A. BARRACLOUGH, Mechanism of blockade of pituitary activation in the rat by morphine, atropine and barbiturates. *Endocrinol.* 57: 345, 1955.

SHARMAN, A. *Reproductive physiology of the post-partum period.* E. & S. Livingstone LTD. Edinburgh and London, 1966.

SHEARMAN, R. P., Ovarian function during and after long term treatment with ovulation inhibitors. *Lancet* ii: 557, 1964.

SHEARMAN, R. P., Amenorrhoea after treatment with oral contraceptives. *Lancet* ii: 1110, 1966.

SHEARMAN, R. P., Investigation and treatment of amenorrhoea developing after treatment with oral contraceptives. *Lancet* i: 325, 1968.

STIEVE, H., Ovulation ohne Corpus luteum Bildung beim Menschen. *Med. Klinik,* 479, 1946.

SURAN, R. R., Ovulation inhibition with sequential therapy. *Fertil. Steril.* 18: 415, 1967.

TAYLOR, A. I., Patau's, Edward's and cri-du-chat syndromes: A tabulated summary of current findings. *Develop. Med. Child Neurol.* 9: 68, 1967.

THOMPSON, M. K., Foetus papyraceous following prolonged hormonally induced secondary amenorrhoea. *Brit. J. Clin. Pract.* 23: 28, 1969.

TORRANO, E. T. and D. P. MURPHY, Cycle day of conception by insemination or isolated coitus. *Fertil. Steril.* 13: 492, 1962.

WATTS, G. F., A. W. DIDDLE, W. H. GARDNER and P. J. WILLIAMSON, Pregnancy following withdrawal from oral contraceptive measures. *Am. J. Obstet. Gynec.* 90: 401, 1964.

WHITELAW, M. J., Delay in ovulation and menstruation induced by chlorpromazine. *J. Clin. Endocrinol.* 16: 72, 1956.

WIED, D. DE, Chlorpromazine and endocrine function. *Pharmacol. Rev.* 19: 251, 1967.

WITSCHI, E., Overripeness of the egg as a cause of twinning and teratogenesis. A review. *Cancer Res.* 12: 763, 1952.

YERUSHALMY, J., On the interval between successive births and its effect on survival of infant. *Human Biol.* 17: 65, 1945.

YERUSHALMY, J., J. M. BIERMAN, D. H. KEMP, A. CONNOR and F. E. FRENCH, Longitudinal studies of pregnancy on the island of Kauai, Territory of Hawaii. *Am. J. Obst. Gynec.* 71: 80, 1956.

CHAPTER III

AN INVESTIGATION INTO THE OCCURRENCE OF OVERRIPENESS OVOPATHY IN THE NORMAL POPULATION

BY

P. H. JONGBLOET, paediatrician*

With co-operation of M. ARENDS, Y. MARGRY and M. STRANKINGA**

INTRODUCTION

Although the actual percentages of mental retardation and congenital aberrations are not known and differ depending upon the criteria used, it is generally agreed that they are considerable. The origin of congenital anomalies and of most syndromes is essentially unknown and one has to content oneself generally with a purely descriptive characterization. Moreover, chromosomal aberrations often give the illusion of providing an aetiological diagnosis while in fact they are only an aid in the description of the syndrome.

In 1939 GEYER analysed 33 cases of Down's syndrome and concluded that the principal cause was fertilization of an „inadequate dysplasmatic ovum". Independently LANDE-CHAMPAIN (1954) concluded that ovarial dysfunction could lead to fertilization of a „borderline" ovum. The discovery of the chromosomal aberration in Down's syndrome, trisomy 21 (LEJEUNE 1959), did not in fact provide any new aetiological factor.

The term „overripeness of the ovum" originated from animal experiments (PFLÜGER 1882, WITSCHI 1952, MIKAMO 1968, and many others). In previous publications (JONGBLOET 1968, 1969 and 1970) it has been argued that intrafollicular and intratubal overripeness might be a causal factor in many cases of spontaneous abortion, premature delivery, still-birth, congenital aberrations and mental deficiencies. The occurrence of chromosomal aberrations in these various conditions would then not be a primary, but only a secondary, and in fact complicating, factor.

* Huize „Maria Roepaan", Centre for observation and treatment of mentally retarded, Ottersum (L.). This article is cordially dedicated to the retiring medical-director G. VAN DER MOST.
** Medical students of the University of Nijmegen.

Fertilization of an intrafollicularly overripe egg can be expected especially during the beginning and end of the fertile age of the woman, or can be due to intercourse after the „mid-cycle", e.g. when applying the calendar rhythmic method. „High risks" can also be expected when factors which lengthen the follicular phase play a part by delaying ovulation. In this respect attention was drawn to conceptions post partum, post abortum, durante lactatione and also after a period of hormonal contraception. Intrafollicular overripeness can also occur as a result of iatrogenic, stress, constitutional, endocrinological, climatological, and viral factors.

Intratubal overripeness, or delay of fertilization in the tubae, can occur in association with the above or as an isolated phenomenon. Such a delay can be expected when fertilization occurs in spite of a low coition frequency, such as in „weekend marriages", in older couples, in incidental meetings and also in the case of the application of the „calendar rhythmic method". Both the lower frequency of abortion (BRUNNER 1941) and of congenital aberrations of the central nervous system (NAGGAN and MACMAHON 1967, HOROWITZ and McDONALD 1969), as well as the higher fertility (CROSS 1953) in (orthodox) Jews compared to other religious groups might then be explained by the application of „niddah". In this practice intercourse is only allowed from the seventh day after the last day of menstruation. Consequently the „midcycle" will be closely approached and the chance of fertilization of an overripe egg will be diminished, since sperm will be present at the moment of follicle bursting.

In a previous investigation of these phenomena, parents of mentally retarded children from our institute were used to furnish starting material. A clear relationship was found between a „positive overripeness anamnesis" and the production of physically and mentally retarded progeny with or without chromosomal aberrations. Consequently, we suggested that the population of an institute like ours is in fact a collection of the results of conception pathology in the normal population. To test this hypothesis, an investigation was performed in a population that was randomly chosen from the towns of Cuyk and Nijmegen.

Although statistically speaking the outcome of this investigation did not always show what was hoped for, the usefulness of the overripeness theory in aetiological thinking could be established. Many unexplained phenomena in human pathology can be more readily understood by it. Therefore we will try to apply it to congenital disturbances in the development of the brain and other organs.

The addresses of 211 R.C. parents were obtained by systematic sampling from the registers in the two towns, Cuyk and Nijmegen. Cuyk has a mixed rural-industrial, and Nijmegen a city population. In Cuyk 120 and in Nijmegen 91 families were included in the investigation. Only two selection criteria were used: the age of the wife had to be between 30 and 50 years and the family had to be registered as Roman Catholic. The age group in question was chosen since it offered a greater chance of finding complete families. Including Roman Catholics only increased the chance of finding couples applying the rhythmic method as means of contraception. After consultation with the general practitioners all couples selected received a letter inviting them to take part in the investigation. No information was given as to the hypothesis of the investigation and complete anonymity was guaranteed from the start, in the sense that the forms would be filled in anonymously. The 211 families were visited in their homes by the questioners (M. A., Y. M. and M. S., medical students). Questions were asked about the circumstances of and the time at which each conception had occurred, disregarding whether the outcome of the resulting pregnancy was normal or pathological. As „normal" were defined children without congenital anomalies and, as far as school-going children were concerned, children that did not have to attend special schools. As „pathological" were defined all children with congenital aberrations, including intelligence defects, neurological disturbances and educational difficulties which made attendance at special schools necessary.

Of the 211 couples selected 56 had to be excluded; 17 because the marriage had remained childless, 9 on account of refusal to co-operate, 20 could not be reached, 5 because the data were untrustworthy (among others suspicion of abortus provocatus) and lastly 5 couples that had produced progeny with inheritable diseases. All these couples were removed from the sample, leaving 155. Assuming that the inhabitants of Cuyk and Nijmegen do not differ biologically from the remainder of the population and that refusal to co-operate or being unreachable did not affect the results of the investigation, we may generalize the data of the investigation for the whole of the Dutch population.

Of these 155 couples the number of normal children was 459; the number of pathological progenies, including abortions, was 122, or 21 %. Because of the written promise of anonymity given to the couples to be investigated, it was impossible to check the information provided by the parents concerning the anomalies of their progeny by means of medical reports. The pathological progeny could be split up as follows:

72 spontaneous abortions (12.3 %)
16 still-births (2.7 %)

34 children (5.8 %) with various defects, given as follows:

   4 children with congenital heart defects
   2 children with congenital kidney anomalies
   2 children with external ear anomalies
   2 children with a non-hereditary thyroid gland deficiency
   1 child with an abnormality of the palate
   1 child with congenital dislocation of the hip
   2 children suffering from Down's syndrome
   1 child rated mentally as an idiot
   3 children suffering from epilepsy
   2 children suffering from enuresis nocturna et diurna (older than 8 years)
   4 children attending a school for the mentally deficient (B.L.O.)
   8 children attending a special school because of teaching and educational difficulties (L.O.M.)
   2 children attending a special school because of severe difficulties in up-bringing (M.O.K.)

As has been mentioned above our purpose was to show that quite a few abortions, still-births and developmental defects might be explained by the over-ripeness theory.

In an investigation of this type the investigator often has to confine himself in connection with the problem being studied. Sufficient information could only be obtained in three investigational groups, which were separated as follows:

1. *Failures during the application of the rhythmic method*

Seventeen couples were found who positively declared that one or more failures during the application of the calendar rhythmic method had occurred. When some doubt existed on this point the couples were not included in the investigational group. In contrast to the certainty of a pregnancy, arising in spite of the rhythmic method, no such certainty could be obtained concerning the length of the ,,safe" period used. Therefore, all pregnancies arising during application of the calendar rhythmic method were included in one group, without separation into those arising before ,,mid-cycle" and those after. This group was compared with a group which will be called ,,control group", and which was formed by all other pregnancies in the same 17 families. The average age of the mothers on becoming pregnant was calculated, since both the application of rhythmic method and increase of abortion, still-birth and pathology might be correlated with the mother's age.

2. *Short intervals between conceptions*

Here all pregnancies from the sample were compared, depending on whether

TABLE I

Number of couples	Number of pregnancies	Pregnancies in spite of application of calendar rhythmic method						Other pregnancies in the same families.					
		Normal			Pathological			Normal			Pathological		
		average maternal age	number	%	average maternal age*	number	%	average maternal age	number	%	average maternal age*	number	%
17	76	32.8	23	77	30.7	7	23	28.1	43	93	20.3	3	7

* age of mother in cases of abortion was calculated using the month of conception.

there had been a short or a long interval between conceptions. First pregnancies of course had to be excluded. In the case of livebirths and still-births the interval can be calculated from the successive birth dates. When the previous or the pregnancy concerned had ended in abortion or a premature birth, the month of conception had to be calculated from the date of hospitalization or from memory. A ,,short conception interval" was defined as three months or less. In the control group all pregnancies arising after a longer conception interval than three months were collected.

3. *Conception occurring prenuptially and during the honeymoon, i.e. in the first 45 days after the wedding date*

It has already been mentioned that the well-known ,,high risk" for the first-born might be due to lability of the cycle in the young woman, to shifts in the ovulation date caused by psychological stress and finally because of intratubal overripeness with the first fertilizing coition (JONGBLOET, 1969). To investigate the ,,stress" factor all first conceptions that had occurred either before marriage or within the first cycle after the wedding date, were compared with a control group consisting of all other first pregnancies. As factors predisposing towards stress ambivalent feelings towards the partner, or towards prenuptial intercourse, or fear for the consequences, or inadequate or incorrect sexual education can be mentioned. It should be noted that the conceptions investigated had taken place before the present era of liberalism in sexual matters.

In these three investigational groups numbers and percentages of ,,normal" and ,,pathological" pregnancies were compared with those of the respective control groups. Wherever possible, statistical analysis of the data was carried out.

Our working hypothesis was that in the three investigational groups described the chances of abnormal progeny are higher than average; that in other words these groups can be considered as ,,high risks". On biological grounds it may also be assumed that these three situations increase the chances of overripeness ovopathy when compared with the respective control groups.

RESULTS

1. *Failures during application of the rhythmic method*

As seen in table I, the same trend is present as in our previous investigation (JONGBLOET 1969). It is significant at a 5% confidence limit. With Fishers exact test the p. turns out to be 3.9%.

52

	Normal	Pathol.	Total
with P.A.*	23	7	30
without P.A.	43	3	46
	66	10	76

* Periodic abstinence.

2. ,,Short" and ,,long" conception intervals

Here again we observe the same trend as in our previous investigation (JONG-
BLOET 1969). The increase in the number of abnormal pregnancies in the case
of short conception intervals, however, is not significant (a one–tailed application of the χ^2 test gives: $0.10 < p < 0.125$).

TABLE II

Number of couples	Number of preg- nancies *	,,Short conception inter- val": ($\leq$ 3 months)				,,Long conception inter- val": ($>$ 3 months)			
		Normal		Pathological		Normal		Pathological	
		Number	%	Number	%	Number	%	Number	%
143	426	27	69	12	31	306	79	81	21

* First-borns are not considered since there is no conception interval in these cases. As 12 couples
had only one child, only 143 couples could be included in this investigation.

3. First-born

Here again there is an indication of the trend which had been noted earlier in a population of mentally deficients, but the results are not statistically significant.

TABLE III

	prenuptial conceptions and conceptions before the 45th day after wedding date				conceptions after the 45th day after wedding date			
	Normal		Pathological		Normal		Pathological	
Number of first-born	Number	%	Number	%	Number	%	Number	%
155	41	77	12	23	85	83	17	17

DISCUSSION

In the three groups investigated the same trend can be found as in our previous investigation (JONGBLOET 1969), namely a relative increase in the number of abnormal pregnancies. Since the groups mentioned concern again situations in which on biological grounds the chances of overripeness of the egg are increased, it may be assumed that in man, too, overripeness of the egg could be a teratogenic factor.

In the same families a significant difference between pregnancies resulting from failures of the rhythmic method and those arising when no periodic abstinence was applied was observed. These results are probably negatively influenced, since also failures occurring just before the „mid-cycle", in other words „optimal conceptions", were included in the investigational group (cf. previous investigation, JONGBLOET 1969 — Category I.A. 5).

Comparing in the same families the average maternal age[1] at conception, it is evident that this is higher in conceptions arising from a failure during practice of the rhythmic method than in desired conceptions. This is to be

---

[1] Data from the Dutch Central Bureau of Statistics from 1961 until 1966 (without 1963) reveal that the average age of the mother at delivery is 29 years.

expected, since the application of contraception is more common after the formation of a full family. However, in cases with pathological progeny the average maternal age at conception is about two years lower than with normal children, showing that the age of the mother can only be partly responsible for these pathological pregnancies. Moreover, in earlier publications it was argued that not the chronological age of the mother by itself is the cause of the relative increase of abortions, congenital aberrations and chromosomal abnormalities, but rather the lability of her hypothalamus-pituitary-ovary system. This lability tends to increase with age, causing the cycle to become more irregular, and possibly lengthening the preovulatory phase, in other words, predisposing to intrafollicular overripening.

Other authors, too, suggest that overripeness of the ovum may occur, during application of periodic abstinence, with malformations as result. INGALLS and BAZEMORE (1969) found, that in three couples who had produced a thoracopagus-twin, twice conception had resulted from a ,,failure during the safe period''.

It has been shown by others that an increase in perinatal deaths follows ,,short conception intervals'' (ROCHESTER 1923, EASTMAN 1944, YERUSHALMY e.a. 1945 and 1956, KNODEL 1968 and JAMES 1968). That congenital malformations and mental deficiency can also be produced in this way is suggested by this and our previous investigations.

Thirdly it is generally accepted that the outcome of first pregnancies carries a higher risk of abnormalities than later ones. In our previous investigation it was clearly shown that this chance of aberrations was particularly increased in pregnancies that had occurred in the first cycle after the wedding date. From the character of the present investigation it is understandable that no information could be obtained concerning prenuptial contacts. Therefore, the group of conceptions occurring in the honeymoon period was extended to include pregnancies that had occurred prenuptially, since it seemed logical to assume that there, too, the stress factor and the chance of intratubal overripeness had increased. Our data seem to point to the same trend as found in our previous investigation. This might be ascribed to lability of the cycle in young women as mentioned before (TRELOAR e.a., 1967 and BRAYER e.a., 1969), but further investigations in this direction would be necessary to establish this.

A number of objections could be raised against the validity of investigations of this kind. The first is that in dealing with a retrospective investigation such as this some doubt always exists regarding the reliability of the data provided. A prospective investigation in these matters, however, is hardly possible, not only from an ethical point of view in connection with the indicated risks of aberrant progeny, but also in practice because of the duration of such an investigation. It should be kept in mind that minimal cerebral disturbances can not be recognized before the age of 5 to 7 years.

Secondly, the fact that only Roman Catholic families co-operated in this investigation does not mean that the conclusions cannot be extended to the total population, since a connection between physiology of ovulation and official religious faith seems unlikely.

A third objection to this investigation could be that minimal aberrations such as educational difficulties and retarded development were also brought into the framework of the ovopathy.We find there is some justification, however, in the analogy with the recorded *seasonal* influence on the frequency of disturbed progeny. Not only mentally deficients (DE SAUVAGE NOLTING 1954, KNOBLOCH and PASAMANICK 1958 and 1960, ORME 1962, 1963 and 1965 and BERGLUND 1967), but also children with partial defects such as dyslexia and educational difficulties (TRAMER 1944, JOHN 1962 and WILLIAMS 1964) are born strikingly more often during winter and summer than in spring or autumn. Many authors also found unmistakable differences in the intelligence of normal children depending upon the season in which they were born (PINTNER and FORLANO 1933 and 1939, GOODENOUGH 1941, FITT 1941 and FRASER ROBERTS 1944). Furthermore, the frequency of winter birthdays among University students is considerably lower than that of birthdays in other seasons (CHENOWETH and CANNING 1941, MILLS 1941). It was argued before (JONGBLOET 1970) that this phenomenon can best be explained on the basis of overripeness ovopathy. This implies that children attending schools for retarded children need not even represent the upper limit of the total spectrum of ovopathy.

A fourth objection, this time directed against the postulates posed here, is that other factors such as abnormal pregnancy and obstetric and neonatal complications, which can also cause developmental arrest and congenital malformations, have not been taken into account. Since, however, we are looking for a connection with a disturbance that *precedes* these complications, the consequences there of can assert themselves both in congenital anomalies of the conceptus and in complications during the course of pregnancy, birth and neonatal period. In a former report it has been argued already that there exists some association between a „positive overripeness anamnesis" on the one hand and these complications on the other. Also, many other investigators have expressed their doubts as to whether the above mentioned complications are the real cause of congenital aberrations and neurological defects. As an example can be quoted the post mortem investigations carried out by GROSS and coworkers (1962, 1964 and 1969) on patients with mental and neurological disturbances. They noted that in 42.8 % of the cases, in which cerebral development disturbances such as agyria, microgyria, pachygyria, hemiatrophy, micrencepahly, etc. were found, the anamnesis made mention of a „birth trauma". The above mentioned investigators, and also PALO and coworkers (1966), who carried out a similar investigation in an institution for the mentally retarded, came to the conclusion that in these cases the clinician had been lead on the wrong track by the anamnesis, since the cerebral disturbances described obviously had not originated at birth, but had arisen at the embryonal stage.

DRILLIEN (1967 and 1968) studied the frequency of obstetric complications in the anamnesis of neurologically disturbed and mentally retarded children. It became apparent that such complications had occurred much more frequently in children that also were suffering from congenital malformations than in children without these. This result, in agreement with general experience, lead this investigator also to the conclusion that much of the total complex of mental retardation with neurological and/or congenital aberrations should be seen as caused by a developmental disturbance taking place before birth. The obstetric complications then are not the cause, but only symptoms with at most only „tertiary" consequences.

Dermatoglyphic investigations in mentally retarded patients whose backwardness was attributed to „perinatal brain damage", too, have thrown serious doubts on the tenability of this „causal" diagnosis. In our institute a similar investigation was performed by VAN ARENSBERGEN and BERDEN (1968). They collected 94 patients that had been admitted with the diagnosis „consequences of perinatal brain trauma" and investigated their dermatoglyphic patterns. On comparison with that of normal populations, significant differences were observed. Since the dermatoglyphic pattern is fixed during the first months after conception, they concluded that already before birth a predisposing factor had been responsible for the „perinatal brain damage" that seemed to have occurred.

Summarizing the conclusions of these different investigators it may be concluded that, as well from post mortem as from clinical and dermatoglyphic investigations, not the *peri*natal brain trauma, but a much earlier operating *ante*natal factor has to be held responsible for many cerebral and neurological deficiencies. It may be asked whether the from minimum to maximum varying phenotypes of mental deficiency cannot be connected to the localization and the degree of deterioration of the egg cell due to overripeness. Quite a number of congenital anomalies, and also of degenerative symptoms or minor defects, could then be interpreted as the „signature of the overripeness ovopathy" in mentally deficients with and without chromosomal aberrations.

SUMMARY AND CONCLUSIONS

By means of an investigation in a randomly chosen sample of the population in the towns of Cuyk and Nijmegen it was shown that also in man over-ripeness of the egg cell can probably be considered as a teratogenic factor. The chance of pathological progeny seems increased in those situations where on biological grounds overripeness ovopathy may be expected. These situations are: 1. ,,failures" during the application of the calendar rhythmic method; 2. conceptions after ,,short" pregnancy intervals; and 3. conceptions before and during the honeymoon. In each of these groups the same trend was encountered as in our previous investigation on parents of mentally deficients. This trend was clearest in the rhythmic method group.

This underlines our warning against the use of the rhythmic method without temperature control, especially in older women or in women with an irregular cycle. It had already been shown by many authors that a short conception interval gives rise to an increase in the number of still-births. Our investigation also showed other dangers for the human progeny arising from a too short conception interval. The lability of the cycle in young women, the ,,stress" factor before conception and the possibility of intratubal overripeness during the first fertilizing coition could possibly explain the increased percentage of abnormal pregnancy products among the first-born. Investigation in the various directions indicated should be continued.

Moreover, the overripeness theory is also useful in clinical thinking, more so than becomes apparent from the statistical data offered, since it throws a new light on phenomena hitherto little understood. The overripeness ovopathy might also explain why the types of mental deficiency commonly ascribed to pregnancy complications, obstetric factors and perinatal disturbances are so often accompanied by cerebral malformations, congenital anomalies and abnormal dermatoglyphic patterns.

SAMENVATTING

Door middel van een onderzoek in een bevolkingsgroep, die aselect gekozen was uit de gemeenten Cuyk en Nijmegen, werd waarschijnlijk gemaakt dat overrijpheid van de eicel ook bij de mens als teratogene factor is te beschouwen. De kans op pathologische progenituur lijkt verhoogd te zijn in situaties waar op biologische gronden overrijping te verwachten is. Deze situaties zijn: 1. ,,failures" tijdens toepassing van P.O.; 2. concepties na een ,,kort" zwangerschapsinterval; en 3. concepties vóór en tijdens de ,,wittebroodsweken". In deze groepen afzonderlijk vonden we steeds dezelfde tendens als tijdens ons vorig onderzoek bij ouders van zwakzinnigen.

Deze tendens was het duidelijkst in de P.O.-groep. Dit onderstreept onze waarschuwing tegen P.O. zonder temperatuurcontrole, vooral bij vrouwen op oudere leeftijd of met een onregelmatige cyclus. Dat een kort conceptie-interval aanleiding geeft tot een stijging van het aantal doodgeboorten is reeds door vele auteurs aangetoond. Door ons onderzoek worden ook andere gevaren aangetoond voor de menselijke progenituur, ontstaan tijdens een te kort conceptie-interval. De labiliteit bij de cyclus van de jonge vrouw, de „stress" factor vóór de conceptie en de mogelijkheid van intratubaire overrijping bij een eerste bevruchtende coïtus zouden het procentueel hogere aantal abnormale zwangerschapsprodukten bij primigravidae kunnen verklaren. Onderzoek in deze verschillende richtingen dient te worden voortgezet.

Meer dan uit deze statistische gegevens blijkt, is de overrijpingstheorie bovendien bruikbaar in het klinische denken doordat zij nieuw licht werpt op tot nu toe onbegrepen fenomenen. Zo kan de overrijpingsovopathie verklaren waarom bij die vormen van zwakzinnigheid, veelal toegeschreven aan zwangerschapscomplicaties, obstetrische factoren en perinatale stoornissen, tevens zo vaak hersenmisvormingen, congenitale afwijkingen en abnornale dermatoglyfenpatronen voorkomen.

We gratefully acknowledge the critical notes made by PROF. DR. T. D. STAHLIE, Free University of Amsterdam, the statisticians DR. E. J. BIJNEN, Sociologisch Instituut van de Katholieke Hogeschool, Tilburg and DRS. M. A. VAN 'T HOF, Instituut voor Wiskundige Dienstverlening of the University of Nijmegen. We thank DR. J. and MRS. G. A. VAN DER MEY, B.Sc. for the translation, and G. PACILLY, medical student for his assistance.

LITERATURE

ARENSBERGEN, J. F. H. and J. H. M. BERDEN, Dermatoglyphen en het perinatale trauma cerebralis. Produced by stencil, 36 pg., 1968. Huize „Maria Roepaan", Ottersum. (The Neth.).

BERGLUND, G. W., A note on intelligence and season of birth. Brit. J. Psychol. 58: 147, 1967.

BRAYER, F. T., L. CHIAZZE and B. J. DUFFY, Calendar rhythm and menstrual cycle range. Fertil. Steril. 20: 279, 1969.

BRUNNER, E. K., The outcome of 1556 conceptions. A medical and sociological study. Hum. Biol. 13: 159, 1941.

CHENOWETH, L. B.and R. G. CANNING, Relation of season of birth to certain attributes of student. Hum. Biol. 13: 533, 1941.

CROSS, R. G., Fluctuating male fertility. Proceedings of the first world congress on fertility and sterility. Vol. I, p. 281, 1953.

DRILLIEN, C. H., *Proceedings of the first Congress of the international Association for the scientific study of mental deficiency (Montpellier)*. B. W. Richards, Michael Jackson Publ. C.L., p. 113, 1967.

DRILLIEN, C. H., *Nutricia Symposium*: Aspects of praematurity and dysmaturity (Groningen). H. E. Stenfert Kroese N.V., p. 287, 1968.

EASTMAN, N. J., The effect of the interval between births on maternal and fetal outlook. *Amer. J. Obst. Gynec.* 47: 445, 1944.

FITT, A. B., *Seasonal influences on growth, function and inheritance*. Oxford, Oxford University Press, 1941.

FRASER ROBERTS, J. A., Intelligence and season of conception. *Brit. Med. J.* I: 320, 1944.

GEYER, H., *Zur Ätiologie der Mongoloiden Idiotie*. Leipzig, Thieme, 1939.

GEYER, H., Die Insuffizienz der Ovarien bei Müttern von Mongoloiden. *Z. Neurol. Psychiat.* 173: 47, 1941.

GOODENOUGH, F., Intelligence and month of birth. *Psychol. Bull.* 37: 442, 1940.

GOUDENOUGH, F., Month of birth as related to socioeconomic status of parents. *J. Genet. Psychol.* 59: 65, 1941.

GROSS, H., A. RETT and F. SEITELBERGER, Ergebnisse vergleichender klinischer und anatomischer Untersuchungen an Zerebralgeschädigten Kindern. *Proceedings of the international Copenhagen Congress on the Scientific study of mental retardation*, Vol. I, p. 451, 1964.

GROSS, H., K. JELLINGER and E. KALTENBÄCK. *Clinical and morphological aspects of cerebral malformations. 3rd International conference on congenital malformations*. The Hague. Abstracts of papers presented. Exc. Med. Found. Amsterdam, p. 45, 1969.

HOROWITZ, I. and A. D. MCDONALD, Anencephaly and spina bifida in the province of Quebec. *Canad. Med. Ass. J.* 100: 748, 1969.

INGALLS, T. H., M. K. BAZEMORE, Prenatal events antedating the birth of thoracopagus twins. *Environ. Arch.* 19: 358, 1969.

JAMES, W. H., Stillbirth, neonatal death and birth interval. *Ann. hum. genet.* London, 32: 163, 1968.

JOHN, E. *The age factor in reading. Retardation researches and studies no. 24*, p. 1, University of Leeds, Institute of Education, 1962.

JONGBLOET, P. H., Overripeness of the egg. *Maandschr. Kindergeneesk.* 36: 352, 1968.

JONGBLOET, P. H., The intriguing phenomenon of gametopathy and its disastrous effects on the human progeny. *Maandschr. Kindergeneesk.* 37: 261, 1969.

JONGBLOET, P. H., Overrijpheid van het ovum. *Ned. T. Geneesk.* 113: 653, 1969. Ibidem 113: 1216, 1969.

JONGBLOET, P. H., Preovulatore of intrafolliculaire overrijpheid bij de mens. *Keesings Med.Arch.* 1582: 8587, 1970.

KNOBLOCH, H. and B. PASAMANICK, Seasonal variation in the birth of the mentally deficient. *Amer. J. publ. Hlth.* 48: 201, 1958.

KNODEL, J., Infant mortality and fertility in three Bavarian villages. *Population studies* 22: 279, 1968.

LANDE-CHAMPAIN, L., The etiology of mongolism. *J. Child Psychiat.* 3: 53, 1954.

LEJEUNE, J., Etudes des chromosomes somatiques de neuf enfants mongoliens. *C. R. Acad. Sci.* 248: 1721, 1959.

MILLS, C. A., Mental and physical development as influenced by season of conception. *Hum. Biol.* 13: 378, 1941.

MIKAMO, K., Intrafollicular overripeness and teratologic development. *Cytogenetics* 7: 212, 1968.

NAGGAN, L. and B. MACMAHON, Ethnic differences in the prevalence of anencephaly and spina bifida in Boston, Massachussetts. *New Engl. J. Med.* 277: 1119, 1967.

ORME, J. E., Intelligence, season of birth. *Brit. J. Med. Psychol.* 35: 233, 1962.

ORME, J. E., Intelligence, season of birth and climatic temperature. *Brit. J. Psychol.* 54: 273, 1963.

ORME, J. E., Ability and season of birth. *Brit. J. Psychol.* 56: 471, 1965.

PALO, J., K. LYDECKEN and E. KIVALO. Etiological aspects of mental deficiency in autopsied patients. *J. ment. Defic.* 71: 401, 1966.

PASAMANICK, B. and KNOBLOCH, H., Seasonal variation in the births of the mentally deficient. A reply. *Amer. J. Public Hlth.* 50: 1737, 1960.

PINTNER, R. and G. FORLANO, The influence of month of birth on intelligence quotients. *J. Educ. Psychol.* 24: 251, 1933.

PINTNER, R., and G. FORLANO, Season of birth and intelligence. *J. Genet. Psychol.* 54: 353, 1939

PFLÜGER, E., Versuche der Befruchtung überreifer Eier. *Arch. ges. Physiol.* 26: 76, 1882.

ROCHESTER, A., *Infant mortality*. Publication no. 119 of the children's bureau, U.S. Dept. of Labor, Washington, 1923.

SAUVAGE NOLTING, DE W. J. J., Considerations regarding the possible relation between the vit. C. content of the blood of pregnant women and schizophrenia, debilitas mentis and psychopathia. *Folia Psychiat. Neerl.* 57: 347, 1954.

TRAMER, M., Frage des Geburtsmonates bei schwererziehbaren Kindern. *Z. Kinderpsychiat.* 11: 11, 1944.

TRELOAR, A. E., R. E. BOYNTON, B. G. BEHN and B. W. BROWN, Variation of the human menstrual cycle through reproductive life. *Int. J. fertility* 12: 77, 1967.

WILLIAMS, P., Date of birth, backwardness and educational organisation. *Brit. J. Educ. Psychol.* 34: 247, 1964.

WITSCHI, E., Overripeness of the egg as a cause of twinning and teratogenesis. A review. *Cancer Res.* 12: 763, 1952.

YERUSHALMY, J., On the interval between successive births and its effect on survival of infant. *Hum. Biol.* 17: 65, 1945.

YERUSHALMY, J., J. M. BIERMAN, D. H. KEMP, A. CONNOR and F. E. FRENCH, Longitudinal studies of pregnancy on the island of Kouai, Territory of Hawai. *Amer. J. Obst. Gynec.* 71: 80, 1956.

CHAPTER IV

MONTH OF BIRTH AND GAMETOPATHY

AN INVESTIGATION INTO PATIENTS WITH DOWN'S KLINEFELTER'S AND TURNER'S SYNDROME

BY

P. H. JONGBLOET[*]

In many countries, both in the northern and the southern hemisphere, the monthly birth frequency of children with congenital aberrations has been investigated. From these data a striking phenomenon becomes apparent: children with congenital aberrations of the central nervous system, facial clefts, stenoses and atresias of the digestive tract, hip dysplasias, and many other anomalies are born more frequently in the winter and, to a less apparent degree, in the late summer. This 'seasonal influence' has already been subject to serious consideration as demonstrated, for instance, by the fact that the *British Medical Journal* has devoted two editorial articles (1958, 1962) to it, in which it was strongly advised that couples who had already produced one child with anencephaly or spina bifida should limit their following conceptions to the winter months as a means of prophylaxis.

The same seasonal fluctuations were found for multiple pregnancies and many other pregnancy complications, for stillbirths, and further for partial defects such as dyslexias and other educational difficulties, for mental deficiency and many forms of psychopathology. An analogous relationship has been recognised by various authors between month of birth and intelligence.

This remarkable relationship between month of birth and congenital aberrations as well as many psychopathological conditions demands an explanation. This is usually sought in factors exerting their influence during the embryonic period, such as U. V. light, cosmic rays, differences in atmospheric pressure, virus epidemics, hypoproteinaemia, hypovitaminoses, etc. On the other hand, PETERSEN (1934), FITT (1941), and MILLS (1941), looked for an explanation, not among factors during pregnancy, but to the effect of atmospheric

The contents of this article were presented at Ottersum on 23 May 1970 at the annual meeting of the Medical Society for Psychiatry and Neurology and the Dutch Society of Hospital Psychiatrists. To be published in *Clin. genet.* 2: issue 5, nov. 1971.

* Huize 'Maria Roepaan', Observation and Treatment Centre for the Mentally Deficient, Ottersum (L), The Netherlands.

conditions around the time of fertilization. HUNTINGTON (1938) and GOODE-NOUGH (1941) believed that genetic factors are responsible for the seasonal increase of these pathological births since 'unfit and impulsive people' are urged more strongly by the climatological conditions to procreate in spingtime. Most of these hypotheses try only to explain the increase of pathological births in winter, whereas the increase in summer is neglected, probably because this was not fully recognised. Moreover, none of these hypotheses has found wide acceptance.

One more remarkable fact seems to us to have been insufficiently emphasized, *viz.* that the maximum and minimum frequencies of the number of births per month of children with various forms of psychopathological conditions and congenital malformations coincide with the maxima and minima of the normal birth curve. Moreover, the similarity between the congenital aberrations indicated and those caused by other 'high risk' conception groups, where overripeness ovopathy is suspected, is intriguing. The increased chance of overripeness of the egg cell has been emphasized (JONGBLOET 1968, 1969, 1970, 1971) for the so-called high risk groups, such as first pregnancies, premenopausal conceptions, and conceptions occurring despite application of the calendar rhythmic method or 'periodic abstinence'.

In these considerations chromosomal aberrations have a very special meaning since nondisjunction can only occur before, during, or shortly after fertilization, but not later. If the same periodic fluctuations in the birth curve also occur for chromosomal aberrations, then the responsible factors must be closely linked to factors which are present around the time of fertilization. If this proves to be the case, then it may be argued that the same factors that are responsible for chromosomal aberrations might also be responsible for various forms of psychopathological and congenital aberrations *without* chromosomal deviations. Such a result, moreover, would partially invalidate all hypotheses which look for the cause only during or even after pregnancy and would support over-ripeness of the egg as an important teratogenic factor.

In this paper the month of birth of patients with three chromosomal aberrations will be analysed: 441 with Down's syndrome collected from our own material and 317 cases of Klinefelter's and 126 cases of Turner's syndrome collected from north-western European countries. As a basis for comparison we have used the birth curve per month of the whole Dutch population.

MATERIALS, METHODS, AND RESULTS

The Birth Curve in The Netherlands
To investigate the fluctuations in the Dutch birth curve, all live and stillbirths per month were recorded over the period 1955–1959 from data provided by

the Central Bureau of Statistics, The Hague. To correct for the varying lengths of the months the formula $(30.433)/x$ was used (where x is the number of days in the month concerned: for February, $x=28.2$). Next, the monthly index was calculated whereby, for the standard index $(=100)$, the average number of births per month over the whole period was taken (see Table 1). In Figures 2 and 3 these indices are set out to make comparisons possible (hatched area).

TABLE 1

All live and stillbirths in The Netherlands from 1 jan. 1955 to 31 dec. 1959

	Live births	Stillbirths	Total births	Correction to length of month	Index "not smoothed"
Jan.	97465	1850	99315	97488.9	98.0
Feb.	93316	1653	94969	102479.0	103.0
Mar.	103906	1777	105683	103739.8	104.3
Apr.	99613	1717	101330	102786.4	103.3
May	103532	1734	105266	103330.5	103.9
June	96693	1568	98279	99687.7	100.2
July	98968	1602	100570	98720.8	99.3
Aug.	98884	1569	100453	98606.0	99.1
Sept.	98927	1560	100487	101927.3	102.5
Oct.	96324	1639	97963	96161.8	96.7
Nov.	91445	1572	93017	94350.2	94.9
Dec.	94391	1610	96001	94235.8	94.8
Total	1173464	19869	1193333	1193510.2	–
Average	97789	1656	99444	99452.2	100

The Birth Curve of Patients with Down's Syndrome

In our institute 441 patients are registered as suffering from Down's syndrome; all were born between 1 January 1945 and 31 December 1968. Almost all these patients were older than one year when they were admitted and/or investigated. This is not an unselected sample of the total population of patients with Down's syndrome. Not all patients with this syndrome in this district are examined by us, and 40 to 60% of children with Down's syndrome die during their first year of life (ØSTER 1953, RECORD and SMITH 1955, BUCHAN 1962).

The age distribution of the patients is shown in Fig. 1. The sex ratio is in agreement with the literature. The patients were divided in groups according to month of birth and the formula above was applied. The indices obtained were 'smoothed' by the formula $(a+2b+c)/4 = b'$ (where b is the index of the month and a and c the indices of the preceding and succeeding month). These calculations are shown in Table 2.

The birth curve of children with Down's syndrome was plotted and compared with the graph constructed for all births in The Netherlands (see Fig. 2).

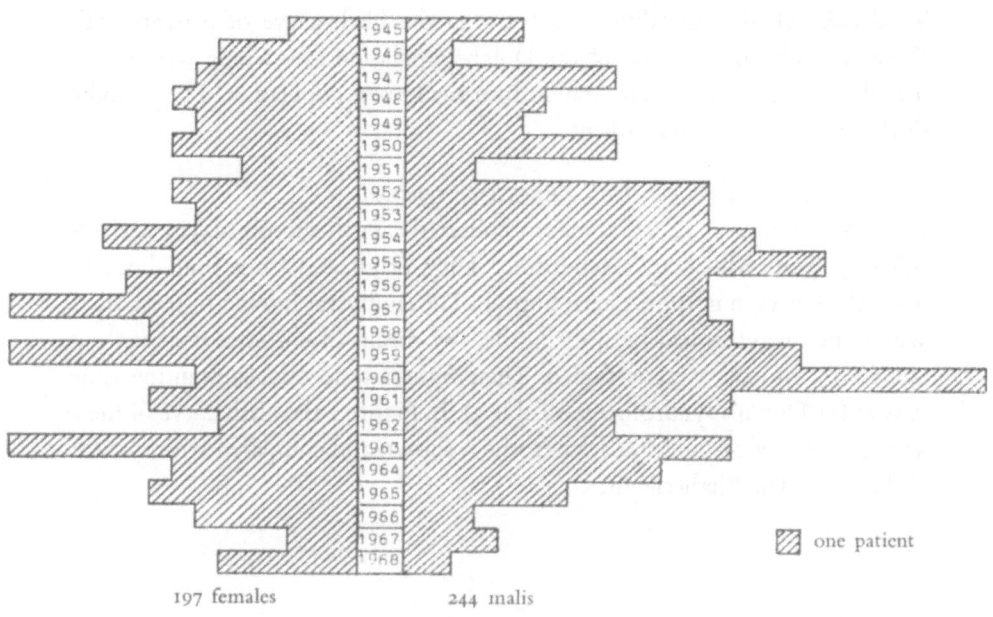

197 females   244 malis

Fig. 1. The year of birth of 441 patients with Down's syndrome.

TABLE 2

Month of birth of 441 patients with Down's syndrome

	Numbers per month	Correction to length of month	Index not "smoothed"	Index "smoothed" by the formula $\dfrac{a+2b+c}{4} = b'$
Jan.	51	50.0	135.9	119.3
Feb.	42	45.2	122.8	120.7
Mar.	38	37.3	101.4	103.4
Apr.	32	32.4	88.0	96.7
May	41	40.2	109.2	104.1
June	40	40.5	110.1	106.3
July	36	35.3	95.9	93.5
Aug.	27	26.5	72.0	84.8
Sept.	36	36.5	99.2	91.6
Oct.	36	35.3	95.9	94.1
Nov.	31	31.4	85.3	87.3
Dec.	31	30.4	82.6	96.6
Total	441	441.0	–	–
Average	36.75	36.8	100	100

To decide whether the difference between the birth curve of patients with Down's syndrome and that of the Dutch population as a whole was coincidental, various samples were drawn from the Down population. The periodic fluctuations were always present.

The Birth Curve of Patients with Klinefelter's syndrome

From the literature we were able to collect the birth month of 317 patients suffering from Klinefelter's syndrome. They originated from four different research centres in north-western Europe. The study was limited to those cases where the diagnosis had been established by means of chromosomal analysis (47,XXY). Mosaics were excluded. These figures were calculated in the same way as for Down's syndrome (see Table 3). In Figure 2 the birth curve of these 317 patients with Klinefelter's syndrome is shown and compared with that for all births in The Netherlands.

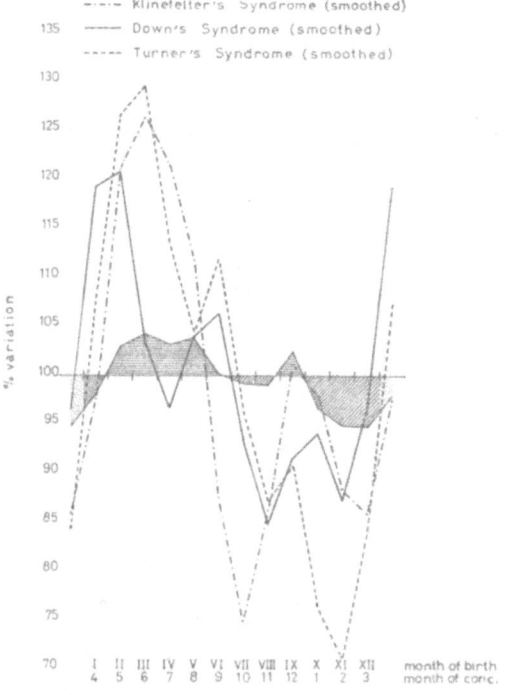

Fig. 2. The birth curves of 441 patients with Down's syndrome, 317 patients with Klinefelter's syndrome, and 126 patients with Turner's syndrome. The curves are 'smoothed' by the formula $(a+2b+c)/4=b'$. The hatched area indicates normal birth curve.

The Birth Curve of Patients with Turner's Syndrome.

From the literature we collected data on the month of birth of 122 patients with Turner's syndrome (45,X; 46,XX/45,X; or structural aberrations of the X chromosome). In the calculations, data from 4 of our own cases are included (Table 4). In Figure 2 the birth curve of these 126 patients with Turner's syndrome is shown and compared with that for all births in the Netherlands.

The Birth Curve of Parents of Parents with Down's syndrome
The month of birth of 318 fathers and 317 mothers of children with Down's syndrome was analysed as described (Table 5, Fig. 3). Statistical comparison was not possible on account of the fact that the samples could not be considered aselect.

PRELIMINARY CONCLUSIONS

A. The birth curve in The Netherlands shows periodic fluctuations (Figs. 2 and 3, hatched area).

B. The birth curves of patients with Down's, Klinefelter's, and Turner's syndromes show periodic fluctuations running more or less synchronously with the general birth curve for The Netherlands. In terms of degree of varia-

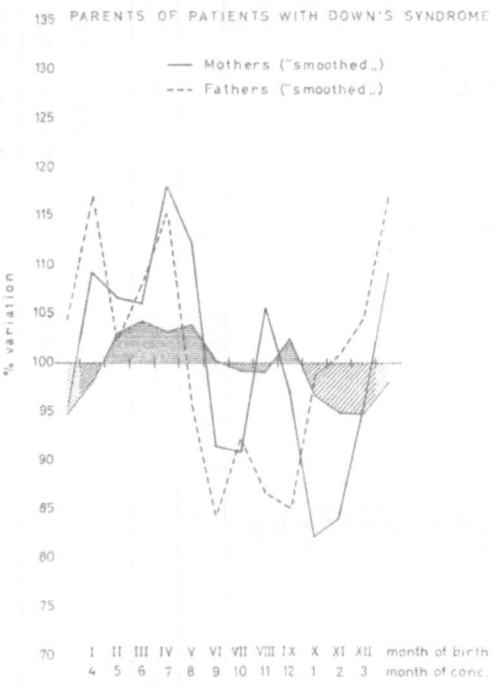

Fig. 3. The birth curves of 317 mothers and 318 fathers of patients with Down's syndrome. The curves are 'smoothed' by the formula $(a+2b+c)/4=b'$. The hatched area indicates normal birth curve.

TABLE 3

Month of birth of 317 patients with Klinefelter's syndrome

	U.K. (Court Brown et al. 1964)	Denmark (Frøland 1967)	Germany (Tünte Niermann 1968)	Denmark (Nielsen Friedrich 1969)	Total No. per month	Correction to length of month	Index "not smoothed"	Index "smoothed" by the formula $\frac{a+2b+c}{4} = b'$
Jan.	9	7	4	0	20	19.6	74.0	97.6
Feb.	14	3	14	5	36	38.7	146.0	121.1
Mar.	8	4	10	10	32	31.4	118.5	126.3
Apr.	5	8	11	8	32	32.4	122.3	121.4
May	9	11	11	2	33	32.4	122.3	111.8
June	11	3	6	1	21	21.3	80.4	87.5
July	4	4	8	2	18	17.7	66.8	74.8
Aug.	5	6	7	5	23	22.6	85.3	86.2
Sept.	6	5	11	6	28	28.4	107.2	100.9
Oct.	6	9	6	7	28	27.5	103.8	97.9
Nov.	10	3	5	2	20	20.3	76.6	88.3
Dec.	10	3	8	5	26	25.5	96.2	85.8
Total	97	66	101	53	317	317.8	100	–
Average	–	–	–	–	26.41	26.5	100	100

TABLE 4

Month of birth of 126 patients with Turner's syndrome

	45,X			Structural aberrations of X chromosome and mosaicism			Total No. per month	Correction to length of month and Index "not smoothed"	Index "smoothed" by the formula $\frac{a+2b+c}{4} = b'$
	Sweden (Lindsten 1963)	U.K. (Court Brown 1964)	The Netherlands (Jongbloet 1971)	Sweden (Lindsten 1963)	U.K. (Court Brown 1964)	The Netherlands (Jongbloet 1971)			
Jan.	5	4	–	1	3	–	13	120.9	107.4
Feb.	4	2	1	1	4	–	12	122.8	126.6
Mar.	3	3	–	5	3	1	15	140.0	129.5
Apr.	1	4	1	2	3	1	12	115.2	113.6

								Index "not smoothed"	Index "smoothed" by the formula $\frac{a+2b+c}{4} = b'$
May	3	4	—	—	1	1	9	83.8	104.5
June	3	5	—	—	3	3	14	135.3	111.9
July	4	1	—	—	3	3	10	93.3	96.7
Aug.	1	2	—	—	4	—	7	64.8	87.2
Sept.	5	5	—	3	—	1	13	125.7	90.7
Oct.	1	1	—	2	—	1	55	46.7	76.4
Nov.	3	5	—	—	1	—	9	86.6	71.2
Dec.	2	3	—	—	2	—	7	64.8	84.3
Total	35	38	2	2	28	21	125	—	—
Average	—	—	—	—	—	—	10.50	100	100

TABLE 5

Month of birth of 317 mothers and 318 fathers of patients with Down's syndrome

Mothers

	No. per month	Correction to length of month	Index not "smoothed"	Index "smoothed" by the formula $\frac{a+2b+c}{4} = b'$
Jan.	33	32.4	122.7	109.3
Feb.	26	28.0	106.1	106.7
Mar.	25	24.5	91.8	106.1
Apr.	35	35.5	134.5	118.1
May	30	29.4	111.4	112.4
June	24	24.3	92.1	91.5
July	19	18.6	70.5	90.8
Aug.	35	34.3	129.9	105.6
Sept.	24	24.3	92.1	97.1
Oct.	20	19.6	74.1	82.2
Nov.	23	23.3	88.3	84.1
Dec.	23	22.6	85.6	95.6
Total	317	316.8	100	—
Average	26.42	26.4	100	100

Fathers

	No. per month	Correction to length of month	Index "not smoothed"	Index "smoothed" by the formula $\frac{a+2b+c}{4} = b'$
Jan.	37	36.3	137.0	117.1
Feb.	26	28.0	105.7	102.3
Mar.	25	24.5	92.5	108.1
Apr.	37	37.5	141.5	115.2
May	23	22.6	85.3	96.2
June	19	19.3	72.8	84.5
July	29	28.4	107.2	92.2
Aug.	22	21.6	81.5	86.7
Sept.	20	20.3	76.6	85.5
Oct.	29	28.4	107.2	98.6
Nov.	27	27.4	103.4	100.7
Dec.	24	23.5	88.7	104.5
Total	318	317.8	100	—
Average	26.50	26.5	100	100

tion, however, the birth curves of these patients seem to deviate from the general curve by a greater amplitude. This phenomenon might provide information concerning the aetiology of the aberration concerned.

C. Analogous fluctuations in the birth curve of the parents of patients with Down's syndrome might offer information concerning possible constitutional factors predisposing to 'pathological conceptions'.

DISCUSSION

Ad. A. The birth curve for The Netherlands shows a broad peak from February to May; a dip during June, July, and August; a smaller peak in September; and a broad valley from October to December.

The literature shows that the birth curve in The Netherlands agrees with those of other north-western European countries (TRAMER 1929, LANG 1931, TIMONEN 1968). A rhythmic fluctuation in the number of births appears to be the rule in all countries, both in the northern and southern hemisphere. HUNTINGTON (1938) calls this typical pattern the 'basic animal rhythm'. Comparative studies show that the moment and the amplitude of 'peaking' in the birth curve may vary, depending upon climatological and geographical factors. HUNTINGTON showed that this birth curve was present in the 19th century as well. From material collected by VAN HOUTTE (1964) concerning all births per month from 1720 till 1755 at LOUVAIN, we were able to construct a similar curve with two maxima and two minima.

An analogous birth curve for The Netherlands had already been detected by BOLK (1902) and WOLDA (1929, 1931). The latter concluded that the birth rate periodicity is gradually levelling off, whereby peaks and dips tend to disappear. He also found that the periodicity is more pronounced in the beginning and towards the end of the fertile age of woman.

The fluctuations described could arise because the day of marriage is seasonally linked. That this has no decisive influence on the birth pattern has been clearly shown by WOLDA (1931) and HUNTINGTON (1938). WOLDA found the same fluctuations not only for third, fourth, and fifth child, but also for the tenth to the nineteenth. On these ground, we feel that the hatched area in Figures 2 and 3 represents the 'normal' birth curve in the Dutch population.

What is the explanation of this 'basic animal rhythm'? An increase in births in winter and late summer could be due to 'pregnancy wastage' of foetuses due to be born in late spring and autumn. This, however, is unlikely, since stillbirths (SLATIS and DE CLOUX 1967) and many pregnancy complications (EUFINGER and WEIKERSHEIMER 1933, PASAMANICK and KNOBLOCH 1958) show similar seasonal fluctuations. It appears more likely that the cause of the increase in the number of births lies in an increase in the number of fertilizations nine months earlier. A comparison with the 'heat' period in certain animals is tempting.

It is well known that rhythmic environmental factors such as U.V. radiation, day-night ratio, and temperature influences have a deciding effect on the 'heat' period. It has been shown, both in the laboratory and in nature, that climatological factors can induce the 'heat' period to occur earlier or later. An example of this is seen for sheep being shipped to Australia. These monooestric animals are in 'heat' in the autumn. In the southern hemisphere, where the seasons are shifted by six months, the 'heat' period automatically shows the same shift. From this we may conclude that the climate exerts its influence on the ovary, where the oestrogens in the ripening follicle are responsible for the 'heat' period.

Some mammals, such as rats, mice, and also primates, are polyoestric and fertilizations and pregnancies are not restricted to a specific season. In these animals regular cycles succeed each other without interruption. In principle, one (or more) egg ripens during each cycle and can then be fertilized. However, these polyoestric animals also show a 'basic animal rhythm'. HUNTINGTON (1938) mentions that rats, even after fifty generations of inbreeding, still show a clear increase in the number of fertilizations in certain seasons, even though these animals exhibit a four-day cycle throughout the year. In the case of domestic animals, which were originally mono- or dioestric, the 'heat' period is often found to have become less distinct. Several breeds of dogs remain sexually interested all the year round but a flare-up of the former 'heat' period can be observed in spring and autumn. This is called a 'latent heat' period.

The two maxima in the birth curve for man could indicate that present day man still has 'latent heat' periods. STIEVE (1950) has reported that Eskimo women are much less active sexually, and even do not menstruate, during the long polar winter. When spring comes, however, they have a period of intense sexual activity. The aborigines of Australia have their erotic festivities in September (when it is spring in the southern hemisphere). Other symptoms of this latent 'heat' period in man could be the pronounced increase in sexual offences, extramarital conceptions, suicides, and urgent admittances in psychiatric institutions during spring (and autumn) and a clear decrease during summer and winter (WILLMANS 1920, HUNTINGTON 1938, CERBUS 1970). Thus man seems to be in a more labile condition psychologically in spring and autumn.

HARTMAN (1932) found that rhesus monkeys were practically sterile during the summer months, and from his data we were able to construct a conception curve with two maxima (a small peak in spring and a marked peak in autumn) and two minima (in winter and summer). This author concluded that the temporary sterility is due to anovulatory cycles. 'Nonovulatory bleedings' during summer were also found in *Macaca mulatta* (MICHAEL and ZUMPE 1970).

Anovulatory cycles are also found in the human female and there are indications that these are seasonally linked. KIRCHOFF (1937) investigated the monthly distribution of endometrial hyperplasia which can be determined histologically by means of a biopsy. He concluded that the frequency of glandular hyperplasia, due to a persisting follicle, showed a curve with a clear peak in the summer. This was connected with an increase in disturbances in the menstrual cycle and in secondary amenorrhea in summer, a finding in agreement with the observations of ENGLE and SHELESNYAK (1934) among young orphan girls in New York City. TIMONEN et al. (1964) plotted the number of conceptions per month in the city of Helsinki against the number of cases of endometrial hyperplasia found in the years 1956 through 1960 in the University Women's Clinic of that city. From the curves it emerges that the peaks of the conception curve almost always coincide with a decrease in endometrial hyperplasia. The rise in twin conceptions in spring and autumn (TIMONEN 1968) also points to quantitative differences in succeeding ovulations.

The foregoing observations can be summarized as follows: The seasonal fluctuations in the conception curve are the result of two basic oestric patterns, a phylogenetically younger with polyoestrus or regular menstrual cycles and a phylogenetically older (mono- or dioestrus). The seasonal fluctuations in the conception curve might be due to alternating periods of normal i.e. ovulatory and disturbed i.e. anovulatory cycles.

Ad B. The birth curves of patients with the Down's, Klinefelter's, and Turner's syndromes show similar periodic fluctuations, running more or less synchronously with the normal birth curve but with a greater amplitude. The agreement between our curve for Down's syndrome and data from the literature is striking. A similar curve, also with two maxima and two minima, may be constructed from the material of COLLMAN and STOLLER (1962, Australia) and STARK and MANTEL (1967, U.S.). A definite seasonal character is evident from INGALLS (1947, U.S.), KÖNIG (1959, Denmark), EDWARDS (1961, Scotland), GREENBERG (1963, U.K.) and LECK (1966, Scotland).

A clear 'clustering' of 'Klinefelter conceptions' in certain months was found by FRØLAND (1967) and by NIELSEN and FRIEDRICH (1969) in Denmark. In the data of Court BROWN et al. (1964, U.K.) and TÜNTE and NIERMANN (1968, Germany) the same phenomenon could be observed. Summarizing the data of the authors mentioned, and using the 'normal' Dutch birth curve for comparison, Klinefelter's syndrome was shown to have a birth curve similar to that for Down's syndrome. Clustering of newly borns with chromosomal aberrations, including Turner's syndrome, was also noted by ROBINSON et al.

(1969) in the U.S. These authors, however, suggest viral-epidemic factors as a possible cause.

The 'Down', 'Klinefelter', and 'Turner' curves show a strong similarity with one another (Fig. 2) and with the birth curves of children with various types of congenital anomalies *without* chromosomal aberrations, such as neural tube defects, facial clefts, stenoses and atresias of digestive tract, hip displasias, many other anomalies, and certain kinds of psychopathological conditions (for references, see JONGBLOET and PACILLY 1971). In practically all these investigations, comparison with the normal birth curve shows that the fluctuations occur at the same time as in the latter but the amplitude is greater.

From the data concerning several types of abnormalities with and without chromosomal aberrations, it may be concluded that definite seasonal fluctuations are always present, synchronously with those of the normal birth curve, but with greater amplitude.

What can be the explanation of this phenomenon? It has been suggested that the seasonal fluctuations in the normal birth curve are the result of two basic oestric patterns interfering with each other. The biological background may be alternating periods of ovulatory and anovulatory cycles. Exogenous factors, clearly influence the mono- or dioestric system. The polyoestric pattern, however, is an autonomous selfregulating system not subject to exogenous factors. A conflicting situation between exogenous and autonomous endogenous factors can be expected at times when both systems exert their influence, i.e. in spring and possibly in late autumn. At that time more than usual interference might occur during ripening of the egg cell with, as a consequence, lengthening of the preovulatory phase or, in other words, intrafollicular overripeness. In this way an increase in pathological conceptions in spring and late autumn would be conceivable and would result in a disproportionate increase in the number of children born with chromosomal aberrations and other abnormalities.

Klinefelter's syndrome is not exclusively due to a disturbance in the oögenesis but may also be caused by aberrations in spermatogenesis. By investigating the Xg blood group, RACE and SANGER (1969) could trace the origin of both X chromosomes in 16 out of 165 patients with this syndrome. In five cases one X chromosome was derived from the father, while in the remaining eleven both X chromosomes were derived from the mother. Generalization of these figures would mean that in about 30 to 40% of the cases, the cause of Klinefelter's syndrome is a disturbance in spermatogenesis and *not* in oögenesis.

It is not impossible that the climatological factors indicated also play a role in the human male. In animals spermatogenesis is also linked and synchronized with the 'heat' period of the female partner. In fish, spermatogenesis is strongly dependent upon light and temperature or a combination of both (SCHNEIDER

73

and IMMELMANN 1969). Consequently it is not impossible that in man, too, exogenous factors may act in an accelerating or interfering fashion, resulting in an increase of meiotic non-disjunction. The duration of spermatogenesis as well as the duration of the transport of the spermatozoon from the testis to the ductus ejaculatorius should also be considered. This may be estimated at more than 64 days (HELLER and CLERMONT 1963) and approximately 21 days (AMELAR 1966), while the whole process of oögenesis in the woman lasts only 14 days. It will depend upon the degree of synchronization of oögenesis and spermatogenesis whether nondisjunction, caused by exogenous climatological influences on the egg cell or sperm cell will occur at the same time or not and thus be distinguishable in the birth curve. In the latter case a two-peaked maximum might be expected in the 'Klinefelter birth curve'. It is not justified, however, to draw this conclusion from the curve shown in Figure 2, since the origin of the second X chromosome of these patients is not known.

For Down's syndrome, unlike that of Klinefelter, no marker gene is available to enable the tracing of chromosome 21 from the father or the mother. Because of the correlation between the occurrence of this syndrome and the age of the mother, the reason is generally sought exclusively in the oögenesis. Nevertheless there is a possibility that patients with Down's syndrome actually consist of two populations, one with the extra chromosome from the mother and the other from the father.

It is possible that the whole spectrum of aberrations due to overripeness ovopathy (and spermatopathy?) can be better demarcated using the birth curve investigation (JONGBLOET and PACILLY 1971). Moreover, confusing combinations of symptoms can be studied from a new angle. Chronically aggressive delinquents, for example, show more degenerative symptoms than control persons (STOTT 1962). They also suffer more often from epilepsy and they have more EEG aberrations, pointing to structural anomalies of the brain (GUNN and FENTON 1969, WILLIAMS 1969). A 'deviant' birth curve, both for prisoners and epileptics as well as patients with congenital aberrations, indicates that gametopathy should be considered as a codetermining factor for these conditions.

Furthermore the association of Klinefelter's and Turner's syndromes with schizophrenia and various forms of oligophrenia might indicate that gametopathy can lead to these deviations separately or to a combination of them. The high frequency of minimal brain damage (OFFORD and CROSS 1969) and of neuropsychological impairment (ROCHFORD et al. 1970) in schizophrenic patients suggests once more the pleiotropic aspects of the overripeness ovopathy as a teratogenic factor. Many cancerous processes, on the other hand, with or without congenital anomalies or chromosomal aberrations (KOBAYASHI et al. 1968, MILLER 1969, MILLER et al. 1969) might be due to the overripeness ovopathy, as the birth curves lead us to suspect.

Ad C. Study of the birth curves for the mothers and fathers of patients with Down's syndrome might provide information concerning the factors predisposing to the production of 'pathological conceptions'. The birth curve for mothers of patients with Down's syndrome has a similar pattern as that for many congenital aberrations. This might support the hypothesis postulated by others that constitutional factors might be predisposing to the conception of a child with Down's syndrome.

Irregular menstruation, impaired generative faculty, recurrent abortions, and an increase in stillbirths and birth of children with congenital aberrations have been noted in mothers of patients with Down's syndrome (VAN DER SCHEER 1927, GEYER 1941, BENDA 1949, ØSTER 1953, LANDE-CHAMPAIN 1954). However, more recent investigations with statistically comparable control groups often showed only slight differences or none at all (SMITH and RECORD 1955, INGALLS et al. 1957, LUNN 1959, BUCK et al. 1965, SIGLER 1967, COWIE and SLATER 1968, MARMOL et al. 1969). In our opinion a wrong approach may have been used in many of these recent investigations. It is, namely, usually required that the control group consists of mothers of the same age group; some authors even require that the mothers in the control group have given birth to their child on the same day as the probands. If the assumption is correct that older mothers have a greater risk of overripeness ovopathy and that 'pathological conceptions' are concentrated in certain seasons, the control groups will obviously consist of mothers with the same circumstances around conception.

Another argument in favour of a constitutional factor in mothers producing children with Down's syndrome is the frequency of 'minor defects' and dermatoglyphic aberrations that can be found in these women (PENROSE 1954, BUCK et al. 1969, PRIEST 1969). ZAJACZKOWSKA (1969) suspected that such aberrations in the mother might be due to mosaicism for trisomy 21. This, however, could not be confirmed by chromosomal analysis of these women.

The average age of maternal grandmothers of children with Down's syndrome is known to be higher at the time of the birth of the mother than that of controls (GREENBERG 1963). This might mean that the birth of a future mother from an elderly woman predisposes to Down's syndrome. GREENBERG (1963) calculated that for a mother below 35 years the chances of producing a child with Down's syndrome doubles if her own mother was older than 35 years at her own birth (0.46 and 0.90 per 1000, respectively). It might therefore be concluded that there is not only a constitutional factor predisposing to having a child with Down's syndrome but also that this constitutional factor might be due to overripeness ovopathy. These mothers indeed are often the product of 'high risk' conception groups (older grandmother and 'deviant' birth curve) and they also often carry the 'signature' of the overripeness ovopathy ('minor defects').

This phenomenon is not strange when we remember the results of animal experiments. One of the first and most important consequences of overripening of the egg cell in amphibians is gonadal dysgenesis along with chromosomal aberrations and phenotypic malformations (WITSCHI 1952, MIKAMO 1968). The birth curve constructed for patients with gonadal dysgenesis points to a similar aetiology. In humans there seems to be a flowing transition from normal gonads (with a normal menstrual cycle) to gonadal dysgenesis (with menstrual disturbances), and gonadal agenesis (with primary amenorrhea). In this way constitutional defects in the ovary might give rise to impaired generative faculty, various kinds of cycle disturbances, and early menopauze.

The 'deviant' birth curve in mothers of children with Down's syndrome strengthens the impression that presence of a constitutional factor predisposes to 'pathological conceptions'. These constitutionally predisposed women might more easily than other women become the victims of interferences of both basic oestric patterns, resulting in 'pathological conceptions'.

The greater amplitude in the birth curve of fathers of children with Down's syndrome is surprising and also more difficult to interpret. Yet in the fathers, too, dermatoglyphic aberrations are known. The dermal index seems to differ significantly from that of a control group (PRIEST 1969). This, too, might point towards a constitutional factor predisposing to non-disjunction. The question whether a subtle affection of the gonads in man might also lead to disturbances in spermatogenesis, causing non-disjunction to be more frequent, cannot be answered as yet. It seems that further research in this direction might be fruitful.

ACKNOWLEDGEMENTS

We have made much use of data collected by G. M. Pacilly, Nijmegen University, during his work at our institute, for which we express our thanks. We are also grateful for the critical remarks of Prof. Dr. T. D. Stahlie, Free University of Amsterdam, and of Dr. E. J. Bijnen, Sociological Institute, Tilburg. The caryographic investigation was carried out in the cytogenetic laboratory under Dr. C. van Kempen, Huize 'Maria Roepaan', Ottersum (L). The tables were prepared by Miss A. M. A. Verstraaten; the figures were drawn by Miss M. Th. Clabbers; and the translation was carried out by Dr. J. A. M. and Mrs. G. A. van der Mey, B. Sc. We thank them for their cooperation.

SUMMARY

Monthly variations in the incidence of births of 441 patients with Down's syndrome, 317 patients with Klinefelter's syndrome, and 126 patients with Turner's syndrome were studied. These three chromosomal aberrations showed almost identical seasonal variation with two maxima, a greater maximum in the period February to May and a smaller one in September. These fluctuations are synchronous with those of the 'normal' birth curve, but have a greater amplitude. To explain the variations, the following hypothesis is proposed: Seasonal fluctuations in the 'normal' conception curve are caused by two basic oestric patterns, of which a phylogenetically younger (polyoestrus) is superimposed upon the phylogenetically older one (mono- or dioestrus). The latter is influenced by climatologic factors. The seasonal fluctuations in the 'normal' conception curve can be explained by alternating periods of normal, i.e. ovulatory and of disturbed, i.e. anovulatory cycles. The increase of 'pathological conceptions' during spring and autumn and the decrease during winter and summer are caused by interference of the two basic oestric patterns. Such interference might retard the preovulatory or intrafollicular ripening of the egg cell, resulting in overripeness ovopathy. In addition, spermatopathy, too, could be influenced by climatologic factors. Birth curves of parents of patients with Down's syndrome may suggest a constitutional factor, predisposing to 'pathologic conceptions'.

REFERENCES

AMELAR, R. D. (1966). *Infertility in man.* F. A. Davis Co., Philadelphia, p. 22.

BENDA, C. E. (1949). Prenatal maternal factors in mongolism. *J. Amer. med. Ass.* 139, 979–985.

BOLK, L. (1902). Naar aanleiding der erfelijkheid van tuberculose. *Ned. T. Geneesk.* 38, 1023–1034.

BUCHAN, A. R. (1962). A study of mongolism in Newcastle-upon-Tyne 1948–59. *Med. Offr.* 107, 51–54.

BUCK, C., G. H. VALENTINE and K. HAMILTON (1965). Reproductive performance of mothers of mongols. *Amer. J. ment. Defic.* 70, 886–893.

BUCK, C., G. H. VALENTINE and K. HAMILTON (1969). A study of microsymptoms in the parents and sibs of patients with Down's syndrome. *Amer. J ment. Defic.* 73, 683–692.

CERBUS, G. (1970). Seasonal variation in some mental health statistics: suicides, homicides, psychiatric admissions and institutional placement of the retarded. *J. clin. Psychol.* 26, 61–63.

COLLMAN, R. D. and A. STOLLER (1962). A survey of mongoloid births in Victoria Australia, 1942–1957. *Amer. J. publ. Hlth.* 52, 813–829.

COURT BROWN, W. M., D. G. HARNDEN, P. A. JACOBS et al. (1964). Abnormalities of the sex chromosome complement in man. *Spec. Rep. Ser. med. Res. Coun. (Lond.)* No. 305.

COWIE, V. and E. SLATER (1968). The fertility of mothers of mongols. *J. ment. Defic. Res.* 12, 196–208.

EDITORIAL (1958). *Brit. med. J.* 1, 695.

EDITORIAL (1962). *Brit. med. J.* 2. 1041.

EDWARDS, J. H. (1961). Seasonal incidence of congenital disease in Birmingham. *Ann. hum. Genet.* 25, 89–93.

ENGLE, E. T. and M. C. SHELESNYAK (1934). First menstruation and subsequent menstrual cycles of pubertal girls. *Hum. Biol.* 6, 431–453.

EUFINGER, H. and J. WEIKERSHEIMER (1933). Der Einfluss atmosphärischer Vorgänge auf den Eklampsieausbruch. *Arch. Gynäk.* 154, 15–32.

FITT, A. B. (1941). *Seasonal influence on growth function and inheritance.* (Educ. Rec. Ser. No 17. New Zealand Council for Educ. Res.). Oxford University Press, London.

Frøland, A. (1967). Seasonal dependence in birth of patients with Klinefelter's syndrome. *Lancet* ii, 771.

Geyer, H. (1941). Die Insuffizienz der Ovarien bei Müttern von Mongoloiden. *Z. ges. Neurol. Psychiat.* 173, 735–741.

Goodenough, F. (1941). Month of birth as related to socio-economic status of parents. *J. Genet. Psychol.* 59, 65–76.

Greenberg, R. C. (1963). Two factors influencing the birth of mongols to younger mothers. *Med. Offr.* 109, 62–64.

Gunn, J. and G. Fenton (1969). Epilepsy in prisons: a diagnostic survey. *Brit. med. J.* 4, 326–328.

Hartman, C. G. (1932). Studies in the reproduction of the monkey Macacus rhesus with special reference to menstruation and pregnancy. *Contr. Embryol.* 23, *Carneg. Instn.* Publ. No. 433, 38–41.

Heller, C. G. and Y. Clermont (1963). Spermatogenesis in man: An estimate of its duration. *Science* 140, 184–185.

Houtte, G. M. A. van (1964). Leuven in 1740, een krisisjaar. Ekonomische, sociale en demografische aspekten. *Pro Civitate. Verz. Gesch. reeks* in-8° No. 3, p. 183.

Huntington, E. (1938). *Season of birth.* John Wiley & Sons Inc., New York.

Ingalls, Th. H. (1947). Etiology of mongolism. *Amer. J. Dis. Child.* 74, 147–165.

Ingalls, Th. H., J. Babbott and R. Philbrook (1957). The mothers of mongoloid babies. *Amer. J. Obstet. Gynec.* 74, 572–581.

Jongbloet, P. H. (1968). Overripeness of the egg. *Maandschr. Kindergeneesk.* 36, 352–366.

Jongbloet, P. H. (1969). Overrijpheid van het ovum. Beschouwingen over de etiologie van het syndroom van Goldenhar en aanverwante congenitale dysplasieën. *Ned. T. Geneesk.* 113, 653–665, 1214–1217.

Jongbloet, P. H. (1969). The intriguing phenomenon of gametopathy and its disastrous effects on the human progeny. *Maandschr. Kindergeneesk.* 37, 261–283.

Jongbloet, P. H. (1970). Preovulatore of intrafolliculaire overrijpheid bij de mens. *Keesings med. Arch.* 1582, 8587–8593.

Jongbloet, P. H. (1970). An investigation into the occurrence of overripeness ovopathy in the normal population. *Maandschr. Kindergeneesk.* 38, 228–242.

Jongbloet, P. H. (1970). Chromosomal aberrations and month of birth. *Lancet* ii, 1317–1318.

Jongbloet, P. H. and G. M. Pacilly (1971). De samenhang tussen maand van geboorte en gametopathie. *Tijdschr. Psychiat.* 13, 198–236.

Kirchoff, H. (1937). Jahreszeiten und Belichtungen in ihren Einfluss auf weibliche Genitalfunktionen. *Arch. Gynäk.* 163, 141–185.

Kobayashi, N., T. Furukawa and T. Takatsu (1968). Congenital anomalies in children with malignancy. *Peadiat., jap.* 16, 31–37.

König, K. (1959). *Der mongolismus.* Hippokrates Verlag, Stuttgart.

Lande-Champain, L. (1954). The etiology of mongolism. *J. Child Psychiat. (N.Y.)* 3, 53–69.

Lang, T. (1931). Zur Frage Geisteskrankheit und Geburtsmonat. *Arch. rassen Biol.* 25, 42–57.

Leck, I. (1966). Incidence and epidemicity of Down's syndrome. *Lancet* ii, 457–460.

Lindsten, J. (1963). *The nature and origtn of X chromosome aberrations in Turner's syndrome. A cytogenetical and clinical study of 57 patients.* Almqvist & Wiksell, Stockholm.

Lunn, J. E. (1959). A survey of mongol children in Glasgow. *Scot. med. J.* 4, 368–372.

Marmol, J. G., A. L. Scriggins and R. F. Vollman (1969). Mothers of mongoloid infants in the collaborative project. *Amer. J. Obstet. Gynec.* 104, 533–543.

Michael, R. P. and D. Zumpe (1970). Rhythmic changes in the copulatory frequency of rhesus monkeys in relation to the menstrual cycle and a comparison with the human cycle. *J. reprod. Fertil.* 21, 199–201.

Mikamo, K. (1968). Intrafollicular overripeness and teratologic development. *Cytogenetics* 7, 212–233.

Miller, D. R., G. J. Newstead and L. W. Young (1969). Perinatal leukemia with a possible variant of the Ellis-van Creveld syndrome. *J. Pediat.* 74, 300–303.

Miller, R. W. (1969). Childhood cancer and congenital defects. A study of US death certificates during the period 1960–1966. *Pediat. Res.* 3, 389–397.

Mills, C. A. (1941). Mental and physical development as influenced by season of conception. *Hum. Biol.* 13, 378–389.

NIELSEN, J. and U. FRIEDRICH (1969). Seasonal variation in non-disjunction of sex chromosomes. *Hum. Genet.* 8, 258–260.

OFFORD, D. R. and L. A. CROSS (1969). Behavioral antecedents of adult schizophrenia. *Arch. gen. Psychiat.* 21, 267–283.

ØSTER, J. (1953). *Mongolism*. Danish Science Press Ltd., Copenhagen.

PASAMANICK, B. and H. KNOBLOCH (1958). Seasonal variation in complications of pregnancy. *J. Obstet. Gynec.* 12, 110–112.

PENROSE, L. S. (1954). The distal triradius t on the hands of parents and sibs of mongol imbeciles. *Ann. hum. Genet.* 19, 10–38.

PETERSEN, W. F. (1934). The seasonal trend in the conception of malformations. *Amer. J. Obstet. Gynec.* 28, 443–445.

PRIEST, J. H. (1969). Parental dermatoglyphs in age-independent mongolism. *J. med. Genet.* 6, 304–309.

RACE, R. R. and R. SANGER (1969). Xg and sex-chromosome abnormalities. *Brit. med. Bull.* 25, 99–103.

RECORD, R. G. and A. SMITH (1955). Incidence, mortality and sex distribution of mongoloid defectives. *Brit. J. prev. soc. Med.* 9, 10–15.

ROBINSON, A., W. B. GOAD, TH. T. PUCK et al. (1969). Studies on chromosomal nondisjunction in man. III. *Amer. J. hum. Genet.* 21, 466–485.

ROCHFORD, J. M., T. DETRE, G. J. TUCKER et al. (1970). Neuropsychological impairments in functional psychiatric diseases. *Arch. gen. Psychiat.* 22, 114–119.

SCHEER, W. M. VAN DER (1927). *Beiträge zur Kenntnis der mongoloiden Missbildung*. Verlag von S. Karger, Berlin.

SCHNEIDER, L. and K. IMMELMANN (1969). Tageslänge und Temperatur als regulierende Umweltfaktoren der Keimdrüsenreifung beim dreistachligen Stichling. *Naturwissenschaften* 56, 93.

SIGLER, A. T., B. H. COHEN, A. M. LILIENFELD et al. (1967). Reproductive and marital experience of parents of children with Down's syndrome (mongolism). *J. Pediat.* 70, 608–614.

SLATIS, H. M. and R. J. DE CLOUX (1967). Seasonal variation in stillbirth frequencies. *Hum. Biol.* 39, 284–294.

SMITH, A. and R. G. RECORD (1955). Fertility and reproductive history of mothers of mongoloid defectives. *Brit. J. prev. soc. Med.* 9, 89–96.

STARK, C. R. and N. MANTEL (1967). Lack of seasonal- or temporal-spatial clustering of Down's syndrome births in Michigan. *Amer. J. Epidem.* 86, 199–211.

STIEVE, H. (1950). Der Ovarialzyklus vom Standpunkt der vergleichenden Anatomie. *Naturwissenschaften* 37, 8–13.

STOTT, D. H. (1962). Evidence for a congenital factor in maladjustment and delinquency. *Amer. J. Psychiat.* 118, 781–794.

TIMONEN, S., B. FRANZAS and K. WICHMANN (1964). Photosensibility of the human pituitary. *Ann. Chir. Gynaec. Fenn.* 53, 165–172.

TIMONEN, S. and E. CARPEN (1968). Multiple pregnancies and photoperiodicity. *Ann. Chir. Gynaec. Fenn.* 57, 135–138.

TRAMER, M. (1929). Über die biologische Bedenkung des Geburtsmonates insbesondere für die Psychoseerkrankrung. *Arch. Neurol. Psychiat.* 24, 17–24.

TÜNTE, W. and H. NIERMANN (1968). Incidence of Klinefelter's syndrome and seasonal variation. *Lancet i*, 641.

WILLIAMS, D. (1969). Neural factors related to habitual aggression. *Brain* 92, 503–520.

WILMANNS, K. (1920). Über die Zunahme des Ausbruchs geistiger Störungen in den Frühjahrs- und Sommermonaten. *Münch. med. Wschr.* 67, 175–177.

WITSCHI, E. (1952). Overripeness of the egg as a cause of twinning and teratogenesis. *Cancer Res.* 12, 763–786.

WOLDA, G. (1929). Interperiodizität. *Genetica* 11, 453–464.

WOLDA, G. (1931). Periodicity, rhythm and symmetry with the births. *Statistical Communications of the Municipal Bureau of Statistics of Amsterdam*, No. 91. J. M. Meulenhof, Amsterdam.

ZAJACZKOWSKA, K. (1969). Palmar dermatoglyphics in patients with Down's syndrome and in their parents. *Pol. med. J.* 8, 1477–1482.

CHAPTER V

STATUS BONNEVIE-ULLRICH AND TURNER'S SYNDROME

OVERRIPENESS OVOPATHY AS A UNIFYING CONCEPT. PART I

BY

P. H. JONGBLOET[*]

Wie oft werden wir über das Turner-Syndrom noch umlernen müssen?

W. LENZ (1967)

INTRODUCTION

To explain Turner's (and Klinefelter's) syndrome WITSCHI et al. (1957) advanced the hypothesis that overripeness of the egg could lead to defective gonadal development. This hypothesis, based on experiments with amphibian eggs, was at first well received (HADDAD and WILKINS 1959). However, the introduction of chromosomal investigations and the finding of many new cytogenetic variants in patients with Turner's and Klinefelter's syndromes pushed it into the background. After ten years now the gains in the field of cytogenetics have not yet adequately explained origin and nosological limitation of the afore-mentioned syndromes.

For, in the first place, attempts to correlate the huge variety of clinical symptoms both in male and in female Turner's syndrome with the equally large variations in the gonosomes have been rather unsuccessful. There occurs e.g. an extreme pregnancy wastage of up to 98% in 45, X embryos on the one hand, while on the other gradual transitions exist from obvious Turner stigmata to normal phenotypes in 45, X individuals. The amount of exceptions is difficult to explain on basis of chromosomal aberrations alone; the latter might be expected to have an all-or-none effect. Moreover, due to the application of karyotyping, shifts in emphasis have taken place. While, in the past, clinical symptoms exclusively served as a starting point for the diagnosis, there is nowadays a tendency to let cytogenetic findings carry the

Paediatrician, Huize 'Maria Roepaan', Treatment and Observation Centre for the Mentally Retarded, Ottersum (L.), The Netherlands.

day. Individuals with an abnormal karyotype, but a normal phenotype, are now diagnosed as 'suffering' from Turner's syndrome, while others with obvious Turner characteristics but with a normal karyotype, should, according to some, be excluded from this group. The latter are now often arranged under another eponym such as 'Noonan's syndrome'. Karyotype and symptomatology thus do not cover each other and consequently the terminology of paediatricians, cytogeneticists, endocrinologists and gynaecologists has diverged considerably.

Intriguing experiments with overripe amphibian eggs (e.g. WITSCHI 1952 and MIKAMO 1968) have been made showing that injury to the egg can give rise to chromosomal aberrations as well as gonadal agenesis and dysgenesis. Evidence, though of a circumstantial nature, has been presented (JONGBLOET 1968, 1969, 1970 and 1971a) that overripeness of the egg can be of importance in human pathology too. The abnormal birthcurve of patients with Turner's and Klinefelter's syndromes indeed points to periconceptional influences, which seem to be intimately connected with the process of ripening of the egg.

It is not unthinkable that chromosomal aberrations are not the primary cause of the abnormal phenotype ('intrachromosomal' theory), but are themselves the result of a far more fundamental process in the egg ('extrachromosomal' theory). One of the arising questions then might be whether there exist gradual differences between the result of inactivation of the X chromosome or its loss. In that case the additional hypothesis LYON (1966) had to add to her 'inactive-X-hypothesis' might perhaps have been superfluous. The Turner phenotype in 45, X women, indeed, was in contradiction with the hypothesis which predicted them to be phenotypically indistinguishable from XX females. Therefore LYON concluded that 'the second X chromosome of human females cannot be completely inactive at all stages of development'. If however, there exist no clear differences between the effects of absence of a gonosome and its physiological inactivation, then the assumption of 'extra-chromosomal' causes for aberrant karyo-, gonado- and phenotype becomes more justified.

It therefore seems worthwhile to investigate whether overripeness ovopathy may offer a unifying concept for the status Bonnevie-Ullrich (st.B.U.) and Turner's syndrome (s.T.), as well as for allied syndromes with and without gonosomal aberrations. To do this we now propose to approach this problem by means of a brief historical review, followed by biological and embryological considerations. In a second part (JONGBLOET 1971c) we shall study by means of fifteen patients the overlapping of the clinical syndromes within this 'spectrum' and investigate their conception anamnesis.

ULLRICH (1930) collected from the literature and from the paediatric clinic in Munich an array of patients with a 'more than coincidental' combination of anomalies, suggesting a possible common aetiology. As obligatory symptoms he mentioned pterygium colli, motor defects of the brain nerves, muscle defects, lymphangiectatic oedema and, as facultative symptoms, hypoplasia of the mamilla, stunted growth, malformations of the external ear, ogival palate, omphalocoele, skeletal anomalies and other malformations. It is important to note that these anomalies concerned boys as well as girls. BONNEVIE (1932 and 1934) suggested an explanation, which was accepted later on by ULLRICH (1936), for the symptoms of the syndrome mentioned. These were supposed to be due to the mechanical pressure of 'wandering cerebrospinal fluid blebs', as encountered in a strain of mice studied by her. Thus the term 'status' or 'syndrome' of Bonnevie-Ullrich originated.

TURNER (1938), endocrinologist from Oklahoma City, unfamiliar with the above mentioned publications, described seven women varying in age from 15 to 23 years, with the following characteristics: retardation in growth, underdevelopment of secondary sexual characteristics, congenital webbed neck with lowering of the hair-line on the back of the neck, and cubitus valgus. FLAVELL (1943) recognized similar symptoms in a man of 21 years and used the term 'Turner's syndrome in the male'.

WILKINS and FLEISHMANN (1944) studied a number of cases of ovarian agenesis, some with Ullrich's, others with Turner's syndrome, thereby connecting for the first time st.B.U. and s.T., which until then had been considered separate syndromes. DANIS (1948) brought congenital ophthalmoplegias, associated with motor dysfunction of other cranial nerves as well as with somatic dysplasias (syndrome of Moebius), into this framework. Finally, CAFLISCH (1952) and WAARDENBURG (1953) added a number of 'Zustandsbilder' showing smooth transitions from one to the other, such as 'dystrophia brevicollis congenita' (Nielsen), pterygo-arthromyodysplasia congenita and status dysraphicus. In this way the Bonnevie-Ullrich-Turner (B.U.T.) spectrum was gradually broadened.

In 1954 various research groups, including that of POLANI et al. (1954), pointed out that Turner patients lacked sex chromatin and 'drumsticks'. At first it was thought that patients with ovarian agenesis possessed a male chromosome pattern. However, POLANI et al. (1956), after an investigation into the colour blindness pattern of these patients, rejected this hypothesis and suggested that they might have an XO karyotype, which was confirmed by various investigators including FORD et al. (1959).

WITSCHI et al. (1957), on the basis of their experimental investigations with amphibian eggs suggested overripeness of the egg as a possible aetiology of Turner's and Klinefelter's syndromes.

The introduction of chromosomal investigations in the years following made that their work received scant attention, however. To be sure, STEIKER et al. (1961) questioned whether some of the aberrations encountered with the syndromes mentioned, were indeed due to lack of a sex chromosome, since typical phenotypes with normal karyotype, such as the male Turner's syndrome, could not be explained on this basis. Moreover, confusion concerning the nomenclature increased, due to the discovery of new clinical and cytogenetical variants and the lack of clear correlations between the two. Symptomatic for this situation was the controversy in the Lancet (1966 i and ii). JONES et al. (1966) complained . . .' as if these contradictions were not perplexing enough, it has been found that streaks are by no means confined to patients with Turner's original syndrome'. They proposed to use the term 'Turner's syndrome' only within narrowly defined limits and to call allied syndromes 'Turner's phenotype', provided they were accompanied by an accurate description. OPITZ et al. (1966) reacted promptly by saying that this proposal was no improvement, 'since individually none of the many anomalies described in Turner's syndrome appear to be in any way characteristic or diagnostic of this condition'. FERGUSON-SMITH (1965) attempted to obtain clearer correlations between karyotype and phenotype by a working hypothesis, the essence of which was formulated as follows: 'the abnormal genotype responsible for Turner phenotype involves monosomy for X and Y homologous loci' (JONES et al. 1966). This attempt was generally accepted and favourably commented upon by many authorities, only to be criticized for the first time by HECHT (1970). As shall be commented further on, clinical observation does not always agree with this basic assumption.

From 1967 on the conception anamnesis of some patients with Turner phenotype led us to wonder, supported by the results of animal experiments done by a.o. WITSCHI (1952) and MIKAMO (1968), whether overripeness ovopathy might not be at the basis of the whole spectrum of B.U.T. (JONG-BLOET 1968, 1969).

2. BIOLOGICAL CONSIDERATIONS

In birds and mammals, in contrast to phylogenetically older animal groups such as fishes, amphibians and reptiles, a specialization into sex chromosomes is found (OHNO 1967). It is generally assumed that two originally similar chromosomes (autosomes) slowly evolved into two differing heterosomes or gonosomes, X and Y. In the male sex in mammals the cell nucleus contains two different sex chromosomes of which the smaller one, the Y chromosome, contains only a minimal amount of genetic information. Consequently, the female, due to her XX constellation, would possess an excess of genetic information, if homologous genes on one of the X chromosomes were not inactivated. This random inactivation of either the maternal or the paternal X chromosome, is called 'dosage compensation'. An analogous inactivation of the Y chromosome in the male is considered a possibility by some workers (HAYMAN and MARTIN 1965).

There seems to be little agreement about the degree of this inactivation in Homo sapiens. According to the original 'inactive X-hypothesis' or 'single-active-X hypothesis' (LYON 1962), one of the X chromosomes is completely inactivated, which implies that both sexes possess only a single active dose of the X-linked genes. The 'complemental-X hypothesis', on the other hand, states that in the female both X chromosomes jointly have the same effect as the single X in the male (GRÜNEBERG 1969). Evidence of the inactivation of one of the X chromosomes is offered by late DNA-replication (allocyclic behaviour) and hetero-chromatinisation ('drumsticks' and 'Barr bodies'). Thus only one X chromosome is normally active and the second (or 3rd and 4th extra) X chromosome is 'inactivated'.

Biological observations show that this 'dosage compensation' mechanism is extremely polymorph. In several mammals it was found that in females one X and in males the Y chromosome is eliminated from the somatic cells (HAYMAN and MARTIN 1965, OHNO 1967 and CORIN-FRÉDERIC 1969). Consequently, lack of sex chromatin and absence of a late-replicating X chromosome in the female is the rule in the genera concerned. HAYMAN and MARTIN (1965) therefore suggested that elimination of a late replicating gonosome during the earliest embryonal stages forms the most extreme manifestation of the 'dosage compensation' mechanism. Conceivably, smooth transitions might exist from euchromatic active stages through heterochromatic inactive stages towards total elimination. Experiments of WELSHONS and RUSSELL (1959) and LYON (1962) with a mouse strain, in which XO females were shown to be capable of normal reproduction, are highly relevant in this respect.

In experimental animals, several authors (KATO 1967, HUANG 1967, RUSSELL 1968, PERA 1969) observed a higher frequency of fragmentations, deletions, translocations and even total loss in gonosomes, than in autosomes. This occurred spontaneously as well as induced by viruses, chemicals, X-rays etc. In Man, too, an increased vulnerability and a stronger tendency towards loss of the late-replicating sex chromosome seems likely, since anomalies of the gonosomes form by far the greatest percentage of chromosomal aberrations. Moreover, in advanced age the Y and X chromosomes are often spontaneously lost without signs of disease becoming apparent (NIELSEN et al. 1969, O'RIORDAN et al. 1970 and PIERRE and HOAGLAND 1971). Late-replicating material of the autosomes, too, seems to be more fragile. At least VAN KEMPEN (1969), by autoradiographic investigation of five patients with autosomal deletions ($46XX$, B_4p-; $46XX$, B_5p-; $46XY$, B_4q-; $46XX$, $E_{18}p-$; and $46XY$, $D_{13}q-$), established that the fragmentation always occurred in chromosome parts characterized by late DNA-synthesis.

To explain the genesis of the s.T. with a 45, X; a 46, $XX/45$, X or 46, $XX/45$, X karyotype (X means here any structural aberration of the X chromosome) the following theoretical possibilities have been postulated (COURT-BROWN et al. 1969):

a. fertilization of a normal egg by a spermatozoön without an X or a Y chromosome;
b. fertilization of a secondary oöcyte which had lost an X chromosome, by nondisjunction or lagging, at the tetrad stage during the preceding first meiotic division;
c. fertilization of a secondary oöcyte, whose X chromosome was lost by non-disjunction or lagging, at the dyad stage during the second meiotic division, i.e. between the moment of syngamy and the fusion of the pronuclei;
d. the loss of an X or Y chromosome in the first or following postzygotic cleavage division; in this case either the maternal X or the paternal X or Y chromosome can be lost.

The possibility a), in which an X or a Y-chromosome is lacking in the spermatozoön is theoretically possible. Its occurrence has often been postulated since it has been proved that in s.T. patients it is often the paternal X chromosome which is absent. However, in this situation the latter could as well have been lost *after* fertilization. We agree that there are no good arguments to reject the possibility of fertilization by a spermatozoön lacking an X or a Y chromosome; in that case the vitality of the ovum perhaps could explain the normal phenotype of some 45, X females.

The possibilities b) and c), in other words the loss of an X chromosome during the first and second anaphase of meiosis, are very well conceivable in the case of an overripe egg, in analogy with results from animal experiments (MIKAMO 1968).

Possibility d), eventually also leading to mosaicism, is compatible with overripeness of the egg (WITSCHI and LAGUENS 1963). The high frequency of mosaics in s.T., (29.6% of the cases according to HECHT and MACFARLANE 1969), and the occurrence of s.T. in discordant monozygotic twins, in which sometimes the karyotypes, in other cases the gonadotypes and still others the phenotypes are different, can, in our opinion, only be explained by disturbances during the first cleavage divisions.

It is generally accepted that structurally aberrant X chromosomes are always late-replicating. They are recognizable by the size of the Barr body. MILLER et al. (1963) interpreted this phenomenon as 'preferential inactivation' of the aberrant X chromosome. Although 'preferential inactivation' never seems to have been proved, it has been accepted without comment. However, this principle is in obvious contradiction to the rule of random inactivation, whereby 50% of paternal and 50% of maternal X chromosomes are inactivated. Moreover, in case of preferential inactivation it has to be assumed that structural deficiency precedes inactivation. However, in mice with an X-autosome translocation, OHNO and CATTANACH (1962) have shown that the abnormal as well as the normal X can be heteropyknotic. Since in this case the structurally deficient X chromosome is passed from parent to offspring and consequently must be present in the egg cell, a preferential and not a random inactivation ought to be expected if the above principle were always true. Therefore, from the finding that structurally deficient X chromosomes in s.T. are always heterochromatic, it does not necessarily follow that the latter is caused by the former. Indeed, both the inactivation and the structural deficiency might be the result of a more fundamental process in the egg or the blastomere.

Connections between cytoplasmatic factors and a pathological course of the inactivation of the X chromosomes are suggested by the occurrence of mono-zygotic 46XX-twins, discordant for colour-blindness (KOULISCHER et al. 1968, PHILIP et al. 1969). Discordancy of X-linked genes in these cases implies dis-cordancy in the inactivation of X chromosomes and, therefore, an exception to the general rule of random inactivation of paternal and maternal X chromo-somes. This exception in monozygotic twins might be ascribed to an exogenous factor. As such, damage to the cytoplasm by overripeness ovopathy might play a role.

On the basis of these observations the following hypothesis can be for-mulated: *Overripeness ovopathy can lead (1) to the loss of a maternal X chromosome a. during the first meiotic division and b. during the second meiotic division, (2) in particular to a pathological course of the inactivation of a gonosome, causing its structural deficiency and eventually its loss.*

The concept that the structurally deficient chromosome is not inactivated or lost by preference, but that on the reverse the deficiency itself might be the result of a pathological inactivation process, demands that the latter takes place very early in development. Overripeness of the egg either occurs in the ovary or in the tuba and therefore meets this demand.

3. EMBRYOLOGICAL-CLINICAL CONSIDERATIONS

a *Gonadal dysgenesis*
JONES et al. (1963) were the first to postulate that *both* gonosomes together are needed for differentiation of primitive germ cells to gonads. There is increasing

evidence that indeed the Y chromosome, together with an X chromosome, is essential for differentiation of the primitive sexual folds into testes. For the differentiation into ovaries on the other hand, neither the short nor the long arm of the second X chromosome seems to be essential, and even if an entire X chromosome is lost a considerable degree of ovarian development can be found.

Although primary amenorrhea is the rule in 45, X women, FERGUSON-SMITH (1965) observed spontaneous menstruation in 10% of these women and BAHNER et al. (1967) even described a 45, X woman who gave birth to a healthy boy who developed normally. In very young 45, X embryos the ovaries hardly differ from those of the 46, XX embryos (SINGH and CARR 1966). In older embryos the first sign of abnormality is an increase in connective tissue at the cost of the primary follicles. In these cases, according to the authors mentioned, the degree of inhibition of development of 45, X ovaries varied greatly from one individual to another. GORDON and O.NEILL (1969), in a similar investigation, often found a normal ovary on one side and a streak gonad on the other, a situation which may be encountered in adult women too. The normal reproductive capacity in a strain of XO mice (WELSHONS and RUSSELL 1959) should be recalled here.

Such smooth transitions from streak gonads to almost normally differentiated ovaries are hard to reconcile with the concept that gonadal dysgenesis is caused by loss or structural deficiency of an X chromosome, for in that case an all-or-none effect should be expected. Moreover, the same variability in the degree of hypogonadism is also encountered in cases of autosomal aberrations (JONGBLOET 1971d) as well as in individuals with Turner phenotype, but with a normal chromosomal pattern. So, for instance, POLANI (1967) mentioned females with a 46, XX Ullrich syndrome but symptoms pointing to ovarian deficiency. VAGUE et al. (1968) pointed to the combination of 'primitive ovarian hypoplasias' and various 'degenerative stigmata' in 46, XX women. Such types of ovarian hypoplasia or dysfunction may constitute the 'marginal' affection of the ovaries, which has been suggested by us as a possible explanation for the fact that some women appear to be constitutionally predisposed to 'pathological conceptions' (JONGBLOET 1971a and d). Menstrual disturbances and a similar tendency towards 'pathological conceptions' have also been encountered in fertile women with 45, X/46, XX and 45, X/46, XX/47, XXX karyotypes (BISHUN et al. 1964, NIELSEN and THOMSON 1968, PREDESCU et al. 1969).

In this respect the ideas of WITSCHI et al. (1957) deserve to be quoted: "Fertilized overripe eggs develop abnormally. Even if only mildly affected, the germ plasm proves highly susceptible to the damage. The primordial germ cells exhibit degenerative features, multiply slowly, and enter the gonadal folds only in small numbers or not at all .In the latter case the animal remains permanently sterile..." and '...The close similarity between gonadal development resulting from experimental overripeness in amphibians and the human types of partial or complete germinal dysgenesis is evident'.

In the male, analogous situations may be expected. In the concept described above, structural deficiencies of a Y chromosome do not greatly influence the building-up of the phenotype. The degree of dysgenesis of the primitive gonads, and consequently the hormonal deficiency caused thereby, will determine the degree of virilization. In the case of agenesis a situation will arise comparable to embryonal castration experiments, in which virilization did not occur at all in spite of an XY genotype. With minor degrees of dysgenesis, fluent transitions may be encountered irrespective of whether the karyotype happens to be 46, XY; 45, X/46, XY; 46, XY; or 45, X/46, XY; (Y means here any structural aberration of the Y chromosome). Thus starting from the normal male, through the hypogonadal subfertile male, the 46, XY Klinefelter's syndrome, the male Turner's syndrome with varying degrees of hypogonadism, the male pseudo-hermaphrodite, the individual with mixed gonadal dysgenesis having on one side an undifferentiated gonad and on the opposite side an ovotestis and, finally, even the female Turner phenotype, are met with. This last type has to be differentiated from 'pure' gonadal dysgenesis which can be considered a genocopy and which differs from the above mentioned syndromes in that it is of familial occurrence, shows no chromosomal aberrations- (the karyotype being either 46, XX or 46, XY) – and, especially, lacks the typical Turner stigmata. 'Pure' gonadal dysgenesis leads to the same conclusion as embryonal castration, since, irrespective of the gonosomes present, it results in the same female phenotype. In extremely rare cases a male pheno- and gonadotype is accompanied by a 46, XX, or even by a 45, X karyotype. The testes in these cases are hypoplastic, although they show definite differentiation. According to DE LA CHAPELLE et al. (1964) their differentiation can be best explained by loss of a previously present Y chromosome. HECHT et al. (1966) indeed found 1% 47, XXY-cells in a phenotypic male with as main chromosomal pattern 46, XX, a case of 'hidden' mosaicism. Consequently, the Y chromosome seems to be necessary for the very early differentiation of primordial germ cells into testes, and further virilization occurs under hormonal control of or induction by embryonal gonads, without further presence of the Y chromosome being necessary.

From the foregoing it may be concluded that the relation between structural deficiencies, or even loss, of an X or Y chromosome on the one hand, and gonadal dysgenesis on the other, is not strictly one of cause and effect. The frequent association of both phenomena suggests a less direct relation of an as yet unknown nature. It is to be expected that studies of the first cell divisions in man and higher animals will help to clarify this point. Such investigations might also adduce direct proof of the occurrence of overripening of the human egg and define its consequences.

b. *Dysplastic developmental anomalies, 'Turner stigmata' and short stature*
FERGUSON-SMITH (1965 and 1969) among others voiced the opinion that the genes responsible for Turner phenotype and short stature are localized on the short arm of the X chromosome and on the long one of the Y chromosome. If such should be the case, monosomy of the short arm of the X chromosome could lead to the types of dysplasia encountered in s.T. and stunted growth. Meanwhile, however, various patients have been described with deletion of the *long* arm of X, but showing in spite of that stunted growth and/or the dysplasias indicated (BOVICELLI 1968, SANTI et al. 1969, HECHT et al. 1970). Even more contradictory to the hypothesis of FERGUSON-SMITH is the fact that similar abnormalities are rather common in the 46, XY male s.T., the 46, XX st.B.U. and in many other complex syndromes with or without chromosomal aberrations. Thus, pterygium colli is often absent in classical s.T., while on the other hand it may be observed not only in patients with trisomy E, or trisomy G, but also in male s.T. and in st.B.U. *without* chromosomal aberrations.

Before the discovery of chromosomal aberrations there was much interest in the 'myelencephalic blebs' theory proposed by BONNEVIE (1932 and 1934), to explain the typical symptomatology. Recently, attention has been drawn again to this theory (LENZ 1967, HIENZ and GROPP 1968, GORDON and O'NEILL 1969). Investigations of abortion products regularly show 45, X and 46, XX embryos with cystic swellings in the neck region and the extremities, monstrous lymphangiectatic oedema and even total hydrops (SINGH and CARR 1966 and 1968, HIENZ and GROPP 1968, POLAND 1968, MIKAMO 1970). In the twenties BAGG and LITTLE and MURRAY and BEAN studied a mouse strain with multiple malformations in eye lids, lower jaws and especially in the extremities. In these regions, where at a later stage the malformations appeared, the investigators had noted, on the 12th and 13th day of embryonal development, accumulations of fluid below the epithelium. These accumulations often remained present right up to birth. BONNEVIE (1932 and 1934) investigated even younger embryos and observed that the blebs did not arise in the periphery, but with regularity in the neck region. She concluded that cerebrospinal fluid had seeped into the periaxial tissues through intracerebral hypertension. These 'myelencephalic blebs' tended to shift from the dorsomedial region to the ventral side, in the direction of embryonal eyes and nose, and via shoulders and back to the extremities. They occurred especially under the embryonal epithelium in folds and concavities and at the tips of the extremities, where they, through mechanical pressure, exerted a disturbing influence on the developing 'Anlagen', resulting in lasting anomalies. Preferential hypotrophy of the left side was ascribed to a slight degree of spiraling of the embryonal axis, in most cases directed to the right, causing a slight difference in the degree of tension of the skin. BONNEVIE suggested that an analogous mechanism in the human embryo might be responsible for the anomalies in the patients described by ULLRICH (1930).

There seem to exist possible connections between overripeness ovopathy and myelencephalic blebs. As a matter of fact, both oedema and various degrees of axial distortion were observed in embryos resulting from experimental overripeness in amphibians (WITSCHI 1952, MIKAMO 1968). It now seems probable that in the human embryo, too, intracerebral hypertension, brought about by axial distortions or other malformations of the myelencephalon, may cause cerebrospinal fluid to leak into the periaxial tissues through the area membranacea superior. A large variety of Turner stigmata could be explained by the resulting subcutaneous accumulations of fluid. In the neck region, Klippel-Feil vertebral anomalies, pterygium colli, displacement of the external ears and cutis laxa might be provoked in this way. In the face, congenital motor disturbances such as ptosis or pseudoptosis of the eyelids and hemifacial paresis might originate in this way, and likewise epicanthic folds, hypertelorism and retrognathy. In the thoracic region and shoulder girdle, absence or dysplasia of muscles, vertebrae and ribs, resulting in various types of malformations may be observed. In the extremities, especially in the concavities of the joints, where fluid blebs tend to accumulate, disturbances in the epiphyses might result in cubiti valgi, shortened metacarpalia or typical knee deformities (sign of Kosowicz). In the palms and fingertips, the most distal accumulation places of subcutaneous fluid, simian creases, asymmetry of dermatoglyphic patterns in the hands, interdigital pterygia, increased digital whorls, and underdevelopment of the finger nails may a.o. be found.

Finally, subcutaneous lymphoedema in the extremities is often the first symptom pointing to a possible s.T. or st. B.U., and lasting disturbances in lymph drainage may be observed in these patients.

However, not all anomalies encountered in the s.T. and st. B.U. can be explained by the 'myelencephalic blebs' theory. Some of them, *viz.* those of internal organs, including the brain itself, must have been caused by factors operating at an earlier stage of development. Stunted growth is a fairly constant phenomenon in s.T. and is therefore usually ascribed to the existing chromosomal deficiency. Extra-chromosomal factors, however, cannot be excluded, since intra-uterine growth retardation and short stature are common phenomena in patients with congenital anomalies without chromosomal abnormalities.

c. Mosaicism and structural deficiencies of gonosomes

It is generally accepted that in mosaicism the phenotype depends on the degree of admixture of normal and abnormal cells in the various tissues, including the gonads. HECHT and MACFARLANE (1969) found mosaicism in 29.6% (154/510) of described patients with s.T. In more than a thousand abortus products studied by others, however, neither a case of mosaicism nor a structurally abnormal X chromosome was discovered. They therefore concluded that selection acts extremely harshly against XO zygotes in the earliest stages of development, and wondered why this might be so. In our opinion equally important questions are why some of the bearers of 45, X chromosome patterns hardly show any Turner stigma, and why on the other hand a small percentage of aberrant cell clones or minimal deletions of the gonosomes are so often accompanied by serious dysplasias. These questions cannot be answered if chromosomal aberrations alone are held responsible for the malformations encountered. If, on the other hand, it is assumed that the circumstances under which conception took place, such as for instance fertilization of an overripe egg, can play a role both in causing various degrees of chromosomal damage and in determining the ultimate gonadotype and phenotype, the problem becomes much more transparent.

ACKNOWLEDGMENTS

We are grateful for the critical remarks of and the fruitful discussions with Prof. Dr. T. D. Stahlie, paediatrician, Free University of Amsterdam and Dr. P. J. Waardenburg, former lecturer in Medical Genetics, Oosterbeek, The Netherlands. The translation was carried out by Dr. J. A. M. and Mrs. G. A. van der Mey, B.Sc. We thank them for their coöperation.

SUMMARY

After 10 years of cytogenetic investigations performed in Status Bonnevie-Ullrich, Turner's syndrome and allied aberrant phenotypes, it has become evident that these deviations are very difficult to explain by their chromosomal aberrations alone. Even if one takes the view that exclusively those individuals should be labeled as suffering from Turner's syndrome who possess the classic XO-chromosomal pattern, then still the chromosomal aberration does not explain the symptomatology. Therefore it is suggested that both the chromosomal aberrations and the various phenotypes collected in the 'Bonnevie-Ullrich-Turner-spectrum' are caused by external factors exerting their influence round the time of conception. As an important factor we then propose overripening of the egg cell. The concept of overripeness ovopathy, namely, offers a possibility to explain the variable and generally rather poor correlations between chromosomal aberrations on the one hand, and gonadotype and phenotype on the other. Also, the concept of 'preferential inactivation' of a structurally deficient X chromosome is discussed. There are reasons to believe that ageing of the cyto- and karyoplasm in itself can lead to a pathological course of the inactivation process, thereby causing structural deficiency and, ultimately, even loss of the gonosome concerned.

REFERENCES

BAHNER, F., G. SCHWARZ, H. A. HIENZ et al., Turner-Syndrom mit voll ausgebildeten sekundären Geschlechtsmerkmalen und Fertilität. *Acta endocr.* 35: 397, 1960.

BISHUN, N. P., M. N. RASHAD, W. R. M. MORTON et al., Chromosomal mosaicism in a case of repeated abortion. *Lancet* i: 936, 1964.

BONNEVIE, K., Zur Mechanik der Papillarmusterbildung, Anomalien der menschliche Finger- und Zehenbeeren, nebst Diskussion über die Natur der hier wirksamen Epidermispolster. *Arch. Entwickl.-Mech. Org.* 126: 348, 1932.

BONNEVIE, K., Embryological analysis of gene manifestation in Little- and Bagg's abnormal mouse tribe. *J. Exp. Zool.* 67: 443, 1934.

BOVICELLI, L., Alterazione morfologica del corredo gonosomico in un caso de disgenesia gonadica. *Minerva ginec.* 29: 1715, 1968.

CAFLISCH, A., *Das Pterygium und sein Vorkommen bei verschiedenen Zuständen multipler Abartungen.* (Status Bonnevie-Ullrich, Dystrophia brevicolli congenita, Turner-Syndrom, Arthromyodysplasia congenita). Leemann AG., Zürich, 1952.

CHAPELLE, A. DE LA, H. HORTLING, M. NIEMI et al., XX- sex chromosomes in a human male. First case. *Acta med. scand.* Suppl. 412: 25, 1964.

CORIN-FRÉDERIC, J., Les formules gonosomiques dites aberrantes chez les mammifères Euthériens. *Chromosoma* (Berl.) 27: 268, 1969.

COURT BROWN, W. M., P. LAW and P. G. SMITH, Sex chromosome aneuploidy and parental age. *Ann. hum. Genet.* 33: 1, 1969.

DANIS, P., Sur les anomalies congénitales de la totalité oculaire d'origine musculaire et en particulier sur le syndrome de Stilling-Turck-Duane. *Ann. Oculist.* (Paris) 181: 148, 1948.

FERGUSON SMITH, M. A., Karyotype-phenotype correlations in gonadal dysgenesis and their bearing on the pathogenesis of malformations. *J. med. Genet.* 2: 142, 1965.

FERGUSON SMITH, M. A., Phenotypic aspects of sex chromosome aberrations. *Birth Defects: Orig. Art. Ser.* 5: 3, 1969.

FLAVELL, G., Webbing of the neck with Turner's syndrome in male. *Brit. J. Surg.* 31: 150, 1943.

FORD, C. E., K. W. JONES, R. E. POLANI et al., A sex chromosome anomaly in a case of gonadal dysgenesis. *Lancet* i: 711, 1959.

GORDON, R. R. and E. M. O'NEILL, Turner's infantile phenotype. *Brit. med. J.* 1: 483, 1969.

GRÜNEBERG, H., Treshold phenomena versus cell heredity in the manifestation of sex-linked genes in mammals. *J. Embryol. exp. Morph.* 22: 145, 1969.

HADDAD, H. M. and L. WILKINS, Congenital anomalies associated with gonadal dysplasia. *Pediatrics* 23: 885, 1959.

HAYMAN, D. L. and P. G. MARTIN, Sex chromosome mosaicism in the Marsupial Genera Isodon and Perameles. *Genetics* 52: 1201, 1965.

HECHT, F., J. I. ANTONIUS, P. MACQUIRE et al., XXY cells in a predominantly XX human male: evidence for cell selection. *Pediatrics* 38: 982, 1966.

HECHT, F. and J. P. MACFARLANE, Mosaicism in Turner's syndrome reflects the lethality of XO. *Lancet* ii: 1197, 1969.

HECHT, F., D. J. JONES, M. DELAY et al., Xq- Turner's syndrome: Reconsideration of hypothesis that Xp- causes somatic features in Turner's syndrome. *J. med. Genet.* 7: 1, 1970.

HIENZ, H. A. and A. GROPP, Zur Genese des Pterygium colli beim Turner Syndrom. *Klin. Wschr.* 46: 1031, 1968.

HUANG, C. C., Induction of a high incidence of damage to the X-chromosomes of Rattus (Mastomys) natalensis by base analogues, viruses and carcinogens. *Chromosoma* (Berl.) 23: 162, 1967.

JONES, H. W., M. A. FERGUSON SMITH and R. H. HELLER, The pathology and cytogenetics of gonadal agenesis. *Amer. J. Obstet. Gynec.* 87: 578, 1963.

JONES, H. W., H. H. TURNER and M. A. FERGUSON SMITH, Turner's syndrome and phenotype. *Lancet* i: 1155, 1966.

JONGBLOET, P. H., Overripeness of the egg. *Maandschr. Kindergeneesk.* 36: 352, 1968.

JONGBLOET, P. H., The intriguing phenomenon of gametopathy and its disastrous effects on the human progeny. *Maandschr. Kindergeneesk.* 37: 261, 1969.

JONGBLOET, P. H., An investigation into the occurrence of overripeness ovopathy in the normal population. *Maandschr. Kindergeneesk.* 38: 228, 1970.

JONGBLOET, P. H., Month of birth and gametopathy. *Clin. Genet.* (in the press), 1971 (a).

JONGBLOET, P. H., Status Bonnevie-Ullrich and Turner's syndrome. Overripeness ovopathy as a unifying concept. II. *Mental and physical handicaps in connection with overripeness ovopathy*, Stenfert Kroese, Leiden, 1971 (c).

JONGBLOET, P. H., Diagnostic criteria for overripeness ovopathy. *Maandschr. Kindergeneesk.* 39 (in the press), 1971 (d).

KATO, R., Localization of 'spontaneous' and Rous Sarcoma Virus – induced breakage in specific regions of the chromosomes of the chinese hamster. *Hereditas* 58: 221, 1967.

KEMPEN, CA. VAN, *Vijf vormen van autosomale deletie. Een klinische en cytogenetische studie.* Gebr. Janssen N.V., Nijmegen, p. 124, 1969.

KOULISCHER, L., J. ZANEN and A. MEUNIER, *La théorie de Lyon peut-elle expliquer la disparité exceptionnellement observée de la perception colorée chez des jumelles univitellines?* C. R. Ier congres int. Neuro-Génétique et Neuro-Opht., Karger, Basel-New York, pp. 242–254, 1968.

LENZ, W., XO-ZUSTAND, Primordiale Keimcellen und Nackenblasen. *Dtsch. med. Wschr.* 92: 983, 1967.

LYON, M. F., Sex chromatin and gene action in the mammalian X-chromosome. *Amer. J. hum. Genet.* 14: 135, 1962.

LYON, M. F., Sex chromatin and gene action in the X-chromosome of mammals. In: Moore, Keith L., *The sex chromatin.* W. B. Saunders Company, Philadelphia-London, pp. 370–386, 1966.

MIKAMO, K., Intrafollicular overripeness and teratologic development. *Cytogenetics* 7: 212, 1968.

MIKAMO, K., Anatomic and chromosomal anomalies in spontaneous abortion. Possible correlation with overripeness of oocytes. *Amer. J. Obstet. Gynec.* 106: 243, 1970.

MILLER, O. J., B. B. MUKHERJEE, S. BADER et al., Autoradiographic studies of X-chromosome duplication in an XO/X-chromosome X mosaic human female. *Nature* 200: 918, 1963.

NIELSEN, J. and N. THOMSEN, A psychiatric-cytogenetic study of a female patient with 45/46/47 chromosomes and sex chromosomes XO/XX/XXX. *Acta psychiat. scand.* 44: 141, 1968.

NIELSEN, J., K. JOHANSEN and H. YDE, The frequency of diabetes mellitus in patients with Turner's syndrome and pure gonadal dysgenesis. Blood glucose plasma insulin and growth hormone level during an oral glucose tolerance test. *Acta endocr.* 62: 251, 1969.

OHNO, S. and B. M. CATTANACH, Cytological study of an X-autosome translocation in Mus musculus. *Cytogenetics* 1: 129, 1962.

OHNO, S., *Sex chromosomes and sex-linked genes.* Springer-Verlag, Berlin-Heidelberg-New York, 1967.

OPITZ, J. M., G. E. SARTO and R. L. SUMMITT, Turner's syndrome and phenotype. *Lancet* ii: 282, 1966.

O'Riordan, M. L., E. W. Berry and I. M. Tourgh, Chromosome studies on bone marrow of three elderly men. *Brit. J. Haemat.* 19: 83, 1970.

Pera, F., Deletion und Translokation heterochromatischer Chromosomen-Abschnitte bei Microtus agrestis. *Humangenetik* 8: 217, 1969.

Philip, J., C. H. Vogelius Andersen, V. Dreyer et al., Colour vision deficiency in one of two presumably monozygotic twins with secondary amernorrhoea. *Ann. Hum. Genet.* 33: 185, 1969.

Pierre, R. V. and H. C Hoagland, 45, X cell lines in adult men: loss of Y chromosome, a normal aging phenomenon? *Mayo Clin. Proc.* 46: 52, 1971.

Poland, B. J., Study of developmental anomalies in the spontaneously aborted fetus. *Amer. J. Obstet. Gynec.* 100: 501, 1968.

Polani, P. E., W. F. Hunter and B. Lennox, Chromosomal sex in Turner's syndrome with coarctation of the aorta. *Lancet* ii: 120, 1954.

Polani, P. E., M. H. Lessof and P. M. F. Bishop, Colour blindness in ovarian agenesis. *Lancet* ii: 118, 1956.

Polani, P. E., R. Angell and N. Polani, Ullrich's syndrome. *Lancet* ii: 421, 1967.

Predescu, V., D. Christodorescu, C. Tautu et al., Repeated abortions in a woman with XO/XX mosaicism. *Lancet* ii: 217, 1969.

Russell, L. B., *The effects of radiation on meiotic systems.* Proc. IAEA Panel, Vienna, p. 27, 1968.

Santi, F., A. D'Alberton and G. Chierichetti, Disgenesia gonadica da delezione delle braccia lunghe di un cromosoma X. *Ann. Ostet. Ginec.* 91: 684, 1969.

Singh, R. P. and D. H. Carr, The anatomy and histology of XO human embryos and fetuses. *Anat. Rec.* 155: 369, 1966.

Singh, R. P. and D. H. Carr, Congenital anomalies in embryos with normal chromosomes. *Biol. Neonat.* 13: 121, 1968.

Steiker, D. D., W. J. Mellman, A. M. Bongiovanni et al., Turner's syndrome in the male. *J. Pediat.* 58: 321, 1961.

Turner, H. H., A syndrome of infantilism, congenital webbed neck and cubitus valgus. *Endocrinology* 23: 566, 1938.

Ullrich, O., Uber typische Kombinationsbilder multipler Abartungen. *Z. Kinderheilk.* 49: 271, 1930.

Ullrich, O., Angeborene Muskeldefekte und angeborene Beweglichheitsstörungen im Gehirnnervenbereich. In: *Handbuch Neurologie.* Bunke-Förster, Springer-Verlag, Berlin, 16: 139, 1936.

Vague, J., H. Serment and B. Blanc, Les hypoplasies ovariennes, leur situation nosographique. *Actual. Endocrin. Journées de la Pitié,* l'Expension scientifique, Paris, p. 127, 1968.

Waardenburg, P. J., Uber retractio bulbi mit Begleiterscheinungen. *Albrecht v. Graefes Arch. Opthal.* 154: 96, 1953.

Welshons, W. J. and L. B. Russell, The Y-chromosome as a bearer of male determining factors in the mouse. *Proc. nat. Acad. Sci.* 45: 560, 1959.

Wilkins, L. and W. Fleischmann, Ovarian agenesis: pathology, associated clinical symptoms and the bearing on the theories of sex differentiation. *J. clin. Endocr.* 4: 357, 1944.

Witschi, E., Overripeness of the egg as a cause of twinning and teratogenesis. A review. *Cancer Res.* 12: 763, 1952.

Witschi, E., W. O. Nelson and S. J. Segal, Genetic developmental and hormonal aspects of gonadal dysgenesis and sexinversion in man. *J. clin. Endocr.* 17: 737, 1957.

Witschi, E. and R. Laguens, Chromosomal aberrations in embryos from overripe eggs. *Develop. Biol.* 7: 605, 1963.

CHAPTER VI

STATUS BONNEVIE-ULLRICH AND TURNER'S SYNDROME

OVERRIPENESS OVOPATHY AS A UNIFYING CONCEPT. PART II

BY

P. H. JONGBLOET*

> *The principal question the nosologist asks is whether syndromes A and B are one and the same entity or separate ones.* McKUSICK (1969)

INTRODUCTION

The monthly number of births in North-West Europe is characterized by a fairly large peak from January to April and a smaller one in September. It was found that these peaks are rather higher for certain conditions, amongst which Turner's syndrome (JONGBLOET 1970 and 1971a). This holds also true for certain aberrations which sometimes accompany Turner's syndrome (s.T.) and status Bonnevie-Ullrich (st. B.U.), such as coarctatio aortae, preauricular appendages, dysplasias of the external ear, micrognathy and anomalies of the extremities (KÄLLEN and WINBERG 1968, MIETTINEN et al. 1970). The hypothesis was developed that these excessive fluctuations could be explained by a rather higher frequency of overripeness of the egg, caused by interference of a phylogenetically older 'spring' and 'autumn' rhythm (dioestrus) and a younger monthly rhythm (polyoestrus). This might lead to both chromosomal aberrations and the abnormal phenotypes commonly gathered together in the B.U.T. (Bonnevie-Ullrich-Turner) spectrum (JONGBLOET 1971b). This approach offers the possibility to present a unifying concept throwing more light on this variable complex of syndromes.

As an example the conception anamnesis will be presented of 6 patients with dystrophia brevicolli congenita (i.e. the combination described by NIELSEN (1934), of the anomaly of Klippel-Feil and pterygium colli), of 3 patients with

---

* Paediatrician, Huize 'Maria Roepaan', Centre for Treatment and Observation of mentally retarded. Ottersum (L.), The Netherlands.

male Turner's syndrome, 3 patients with non-familial syndrome of Möbius, and finally 3 patients with monosomy of the X-chromosome. The first three syndromes had already been connected with the st. B.U. before the chromosomal era, namely dystrophia brevicolli congenita by CAFLISCH in 1952, male Turner's syndrome by FLAVELL in 1943, and the syndrome of Möbius by DANIS in 1948. The fourth group with monosomy of X is integrated in this spectrum by its cytogenetic aspects.

One of the patients with short neck and Klippel-Feil anomaly (no. 5, see Table) was described in a previous publication (JONGBLOET 1968). She also had dermolipoids of the limbus corneae and auricular appendages, a combination of symptoms known as Goldenhar's syndrome. It should be noted that, before GOLDENHAR described it under the name of oculo-auriculo-vertebral syndrome (1952), this complex of symptoms had been included in the st. B.U. by COTTERMAN and FALLS (1949). Another patient with brevicollis and Klippel-Feil anomaly is a mongoloid girl with classical trisomy G. The first to describe the association of Down's syndrome with pterygium colli in two patients was ULLRICH in his original publication (1930).

MODE OF INVESTIGATION

The patients with brevicollis and Klippel-Feil anomaly, with male Turner syndrome and with non-familial Möbius' syndrome were selected on their clinical appearance. The pedigree of the latter was explored to the sixth generation, to ensure that there indeed existed no consanguinity.

The three females with absence or near-absence of sex chromatin were found by studying the Barr-bodies, an investigation routinely done in all our patients. Moreover, all patients underwent a thorough cytogenetical clinical and psychological examination. A profound hetero-anamnesis was taken concerning these patients, with special attention to the circumstances around conception. It should be stressed that the patients were selected first, and that the conception anamnesis was taken thereafter, to prevent bias. The pertinent data are arranged in Table I, II and III; the photographs show the patients' outward appearance.

DISCUSSION OF THE FINDINGS

Previous investigations had made it probable that conceptions occurring under certain circumstances run an abnormally high risk of resulting either in a non-viable conceptus or a malformed or handicapped child. To explain this it was hypothesized that these circumstances might easily lead to overripening of the ovum before fertilization (JONGBLOET 1969, 1970, 1971a). It was further argued that this might be one of the main causes of certain non-familial connatal abnormalities, such as the B.U.T. spectrum in all its varieties (JONGBLOET 1971b). The purpose of the present investigation was to test this hypothesis by conducting a retrospective study of the circumstances under which conception had occurred, in a number of patients who, on clinical grounds, 'belong' to this spectrum. As can be seen from Table 1, the conception anamnesis is suspect for overripeness ovopathy in 13 out of the 15 cases. Only in cases 2 and 4 the circumstances round the conception seemed to be entirely normal. Frequently a number of factors which could have reinforced each other were encountered.

Two mothers (nos. 9 and 12) had been older than 40 years at the time of conception. In three mothers (nos. 5, 9 and 10) the conception interval was very short and in a fourth (no. 1) a post-partum oligomenorrhea was mentioned, complicated by treatment for hypertension (Reserpine® $3 \times \frac{1}{4}$ mgs. dd.) and adipositas (Pentoadiparthrol® 0.013 gms dd., a pentobarbiturate of D-amphetamine). In case no. 6 the mother had also been treated for hypertension but the nature of the drug could not be ascertained.

Six couples found themselves with a pregnancy in spite of applying the calendar rhythmic method. In two of these (nos. 1 and 4) the menstrual cycle was reported as still being irregular after the preceding delivery. In a third case (no. 12) the woman had been 41 years old, and a fourth (no. 15) informed us that her cycle had always been irregular. The mother of patient no. 8 had observed that the menstruation was still 'pushing through' when to her surprise she felt 'she was already pregnant and vomiting'. Her suspicion was confirmed when child movements started already at $3\frac{1}{2}$ months after the 'last supposed menstruation' and birth occurred after '8 months', while the birth weight was approximately ± 3.500 gms. This might be a typical example of 'high birth weight-low gestational age'. The mother of patient no. 7 had wanted to become pregnant but, after a miscarriage, six months of 'severe periodic abstinence' were prescribed and carried into effect by the parents. Yet conception must have taken place before the end of this period, since only 8 months after discontinuing abstinence a child of approx. 3.000 gms. was born.

In two women endocrinological disturbances were present at the moment of conception. In case no. 3 hypothyroidy had been suspected, but left untreated. During this period first a miscarriage and, following that, the pregnancy concerned had occurred. Only after delivery the diagnosis of hypothyroidy had been confirmed (P.B.I.: 1,2 mg/100 ml.), and treatment had been started with 75 mgs. of Thyranon® per day, after which the clinical symptoms had disappeared. The second woman (no. 13) had been treated with an 'insulin fattening cure' on account of abnormal thinness. Irregular cycles ascribed to this cure were treated by a gynaecologist with Duphaston® (10 mgs. daily). A few weeks later however, she had become pregnant against her wish.

Finally, climatological circumstances may also have played a part. It should

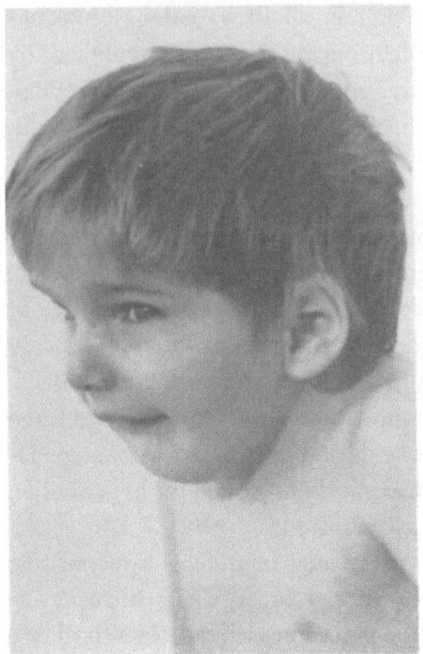

Patient no. 1

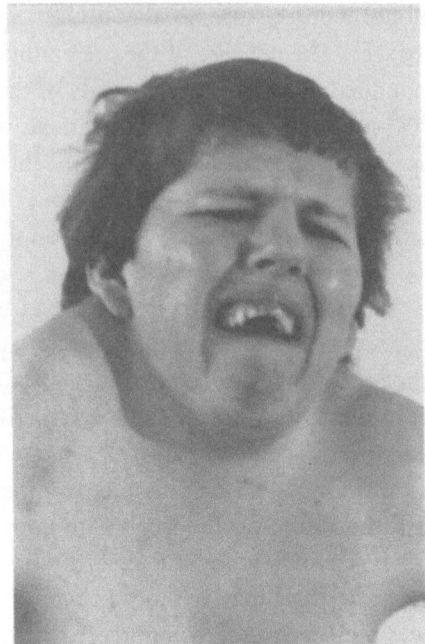

Patient no. 2

Patient no. 3

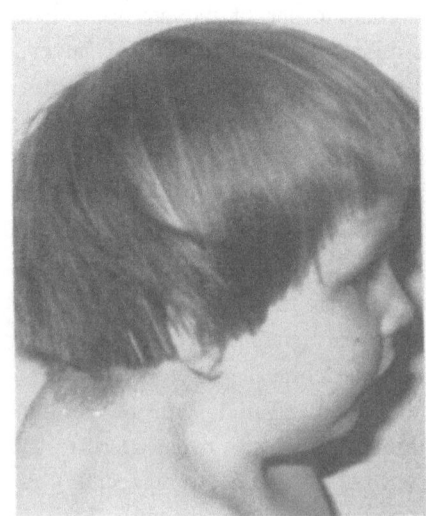

Patients no. 1, 2, 3, 4, 5 and 6.

Patients with dystrophia brevicollis congenita (Klippel-Feil anomaly and pterygium colli). Patient no. 5 has all the symptoms of Goldenhar's syndrome and patient no. 6 shows trisomy G.

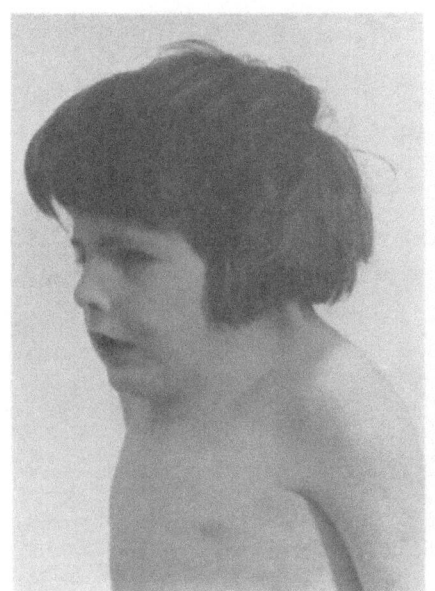
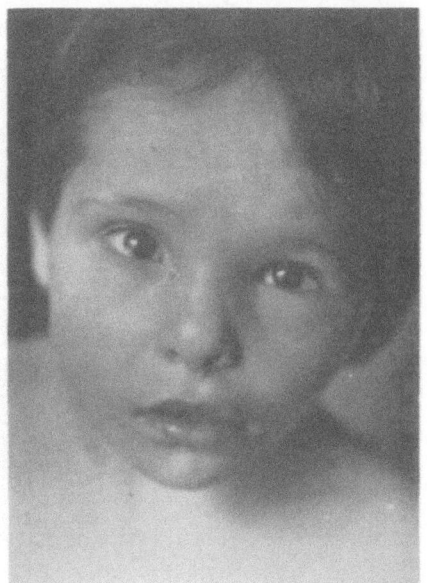

Patient no. 4

Patient no. 5

Patient no. 6

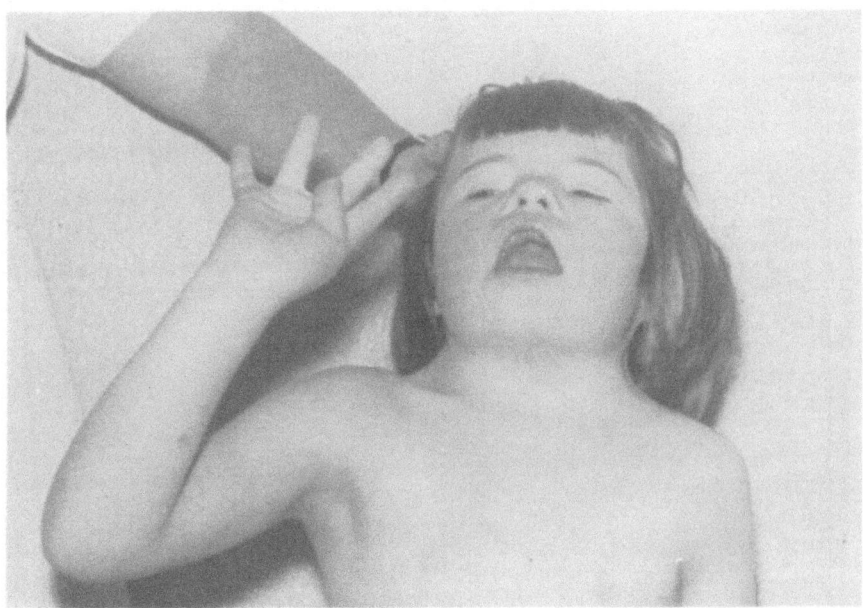

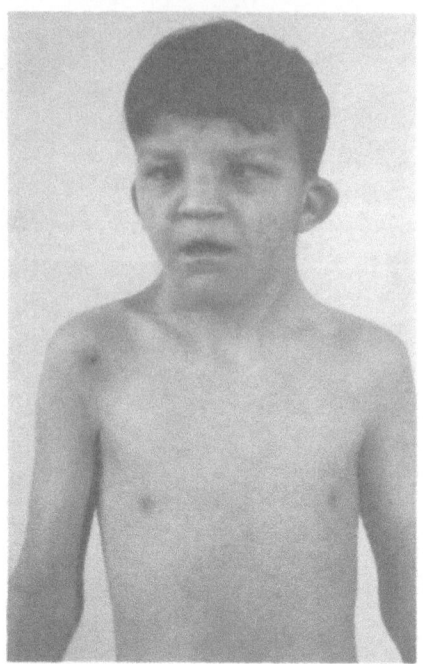

Patient no. 7

Patient no. 8

Patient no. 9

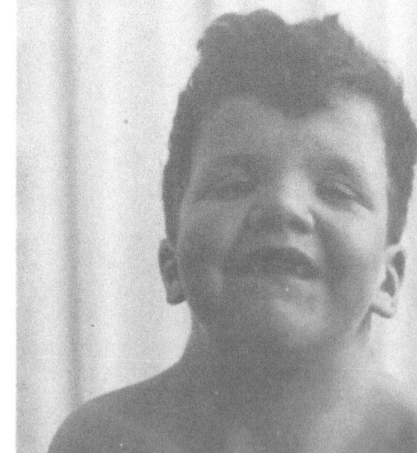

Patients no. 7, 8 and 9.
Patients with male Turner's syndrome, the karyotype being 46, XY.

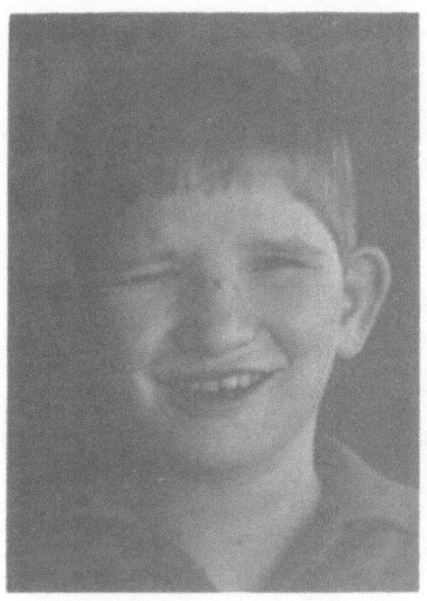

Patient no. 10

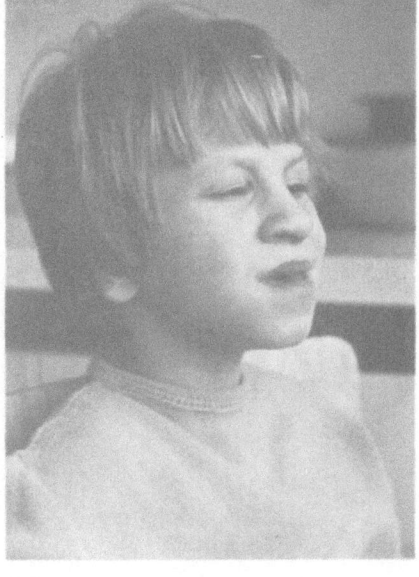

Patient no. 11

Patient no. 12
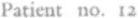

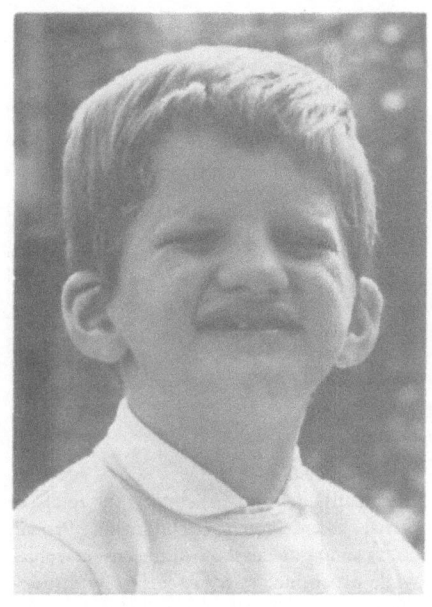

Patients no, 10, 11 and 12.

Patients with non-familial syndrome of Möbius, with striking impairment of motor function of cranial nerves, and various Turner stigmata. Patient no. 12 shows (presumably) an isochromosome of the long arms of X.

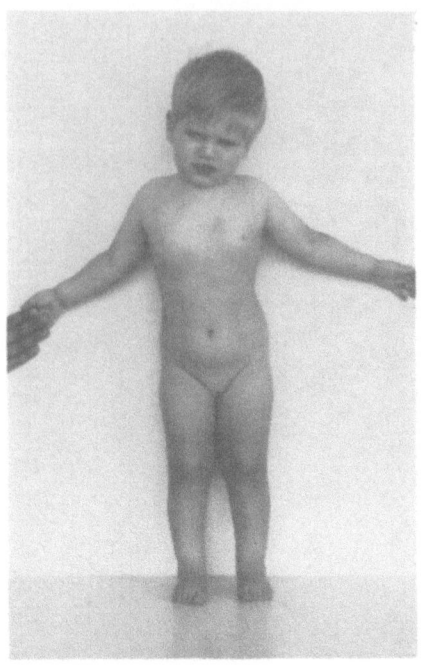

Patient no. 13

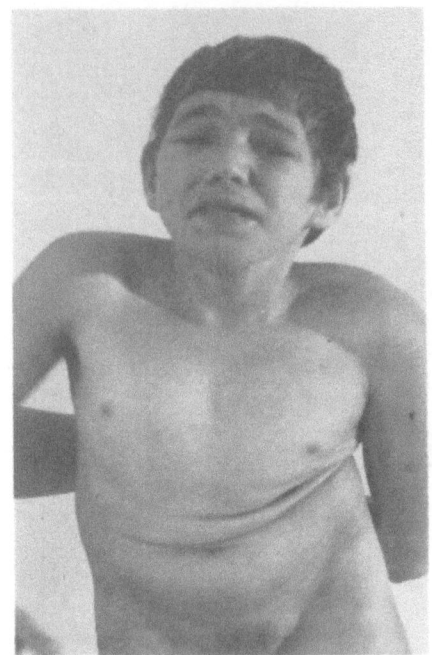

Patient no. 14

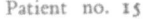

Patient no. 15

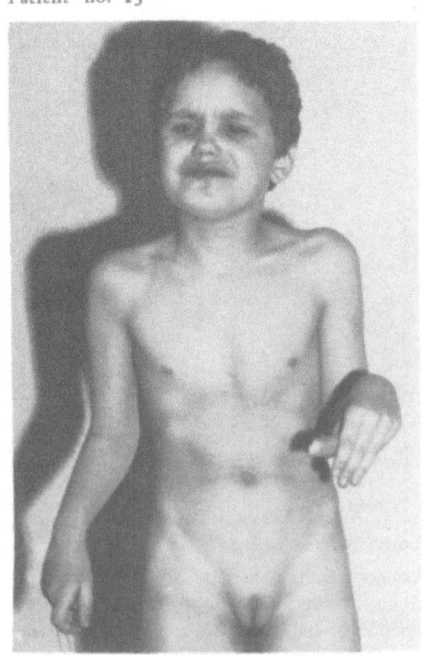

Patients no. 13, 14 and 15.

Apparently female patients with total or partial absence of sex chromatin. Patients no. 13 and 15 do not show distinct dysmorphias, while patient no. 14 is extremely dysplastic.

be noted that 12 of the 15 patients had been born in the 'high risk' months, being the four first months of the year, and August and September (JONGBLOET 1971a). No statistically reliable conclusion, however, can be drawn from these small numbers.

Table II shows a distinct increase of pregnancy wastage in the mothers and of multiple births and congenital malformations in the sibships. Furthermore, there seems to be a marked rise of complications during pregnancy, parturition and neonatal life of the propositi.

GENERAL DISCUSSION

The circumstances which might lead to delayed ovulation and/or fertilization of the egg have been thoroughly discussed elsewhere (JONGBLOET 1969, 1970, 1971a). That in the majority of these patients, selected on clinical and cytogenetic grounds, circumstances predisposing towards overripeness of the egg were found, might be conducive towards a better understanding of (1) the overlapping of symptoms in the various syndromes which can be included in the B.U.T. spectrum and (2) the highly variable symptomatology. Finally, (3) a 'positive overripeness anamnesis' might be a useful criterion to distinguish between these syndromes and those of genetic origin.

1. Overripeness ovopathy as an aetiologically unifying concept can explain why demarcation of the various syndromes incorporated in the B.U.T. spectrum is so difficult.

In the presentation of the patients, the association between Goldenhar's, respectively Down's syndrome and dystrophia brevicolli congenita has been pointed out. Within the groups mentioned other demarcations, too, proved to be very difficult. Patient no. 10, for instance, classified as having Möbius' syndrome, might as well be included in the group with male Turner's syndrome, on account of the low hair line, low-set ears, thoracic anomaly, polythely and increased gonadotrophin secretion. Patient no. 12, also with Möbius' syndrome, presumably possessed an isochromosome of the long arms of X (46, XXqi). This patient therefore might also be placed with those showing abnormalities of the X chromosome.

Various other syndromes, too, show relations with the st. B.U. and can be brought under the same aetiological denominator, *viz.* overripeness ovopathy. So, for instance, a child with unilateral muscle defects of the thorax and homolateral malformations of the hand (so-called Poland's syndrome) had been conceived during post-partum amenorrhea complicated by treatment with psychopharmaca (GORDON 1970).

Table I

Number of patient	Number of registration	Date of birth	Criterion of selection	Phenotype	Karyotype	Sex-chromatin	Sibship	Peculiarities concerning sibship
1	1471	17–9–'65	KLIPPEL-FEIL and PTERYGIUM COLLI	♀	46,XX	pos.		no. 2 is operated for spina bifida occulta
2	320	8–8–'50	KLIPPEL-FEIL and PTERYGIUM COLLI	♀	46,XX	pos.		
3	897	3–8–'58	KLIPPEL-FEIL and PTERYGIUM COLLI	♀	46,XX	pos.		
4	1337	7–5–'64	KLIPPEL-FEIL and PTERYGIUM COLLI	♀	46,XX	pos.		no. 1: meningomyelocele
5	1026	13–1–'63	KLIPPEL-FEIL and PTERYGIUM COLLI	♀	46,XX	pos.		no. 3: operated for ureter obstruction
6	779	30–6–'56	KLIPPEL-FEIL and PTERYGIUM COLLI	♀	47,XXG	pos.		
7	511	25–2–'57	MALE TURNER SYNDROME	♂	46,XY	neg.		
8	1232	14–3–'62	MALE TURNER SYNDROME	♂	46,XY	neg.		
9	1523	4–6–'62	MALE TURNER SYNDROME	♂	46,XY	neg.		no. 1+2: neonatal death; no. 5: died from diphteria; no. 8: nystagmus; no. 10: neurologic disturb
10	629	17–3–'56	NON FAMILIAL MÖBIUS SYNDROME	♂	46,XY	neg.		no consanguinity (6 generations)
11	1065	8–9–'58	NON FAMILIAL MÖBIUS SYNDROME	♀	46,XX	pos.		no consanguinity (6 generations) no. 3: neurologic disturb. no. 5: foetus maceratus
12	1176	3–4–'62	NON FAMILIAL MÖBIUS SYNDROME	♀	46,XXqi	pos.		no consanguinity (6 generations)
13	1270	3–3–'66	DECREASE OF SEX-CHROMATIN	♀	45,X/46,XXq+	neg./pos.		
14	172	16–4–'45	ABSENCE OF SEX-CHROMATIN	♀	45,X	neg.		
15	1228	3–2–'61	ABSENCE OF SEX-CHROMATIN	♀	45,X	neg.		

abortions	18
cong. malformations 6+15 prop.	
still births	3
twin births	2
total of pregnancies	94
without propositi	79

In no family, identical malformations were known

⊠ ⊗ dead
▲ spontaneous abortion
■ ● propositi
◪ ◐ congenital defect

Circumstances around conception of propositi	End of reproductive period	Short conception interval	Long unintended conception-interval	Endocrinological disturbances	'Spring' and 'autumn' conceptions	Failures during practice of C.R.M.*	during pharmacological treatment	Age at birth mother	father	Parity
failure during practice of C.R.M.*, during post partum oligomenorrhea and treatment with reserpine 3×¼ mgr. (hypertension) and pento-adiparthrol ® (adipositas)					+	+	+	30 4	34 9	7/8
					+			34.1	33.9	2/2
hypothyroidy: P.B.I.; 1, 2 mgr./100 ml. after birth: R/75 mgr. thyranon ®				+	+			28 1	30 10	3/3
								32 9	30.8	3/4
failure during practice of C.R.M.*, post partum.		+			+	+		34.10	36.5	6/7
failure during pharmacological treatment for hypertension (reserpine ?)							+	35.1	33.11	5/5
'accidental pregnancy' before the end of a period of prescribed C.R.M.*					+	+		39.9	38.0	3/3
failure during practice of C.R.M.*					+	+		33.9	37.1	6/7
conception preceded by two abortions within 5 months.	+	+						42.11	49.9	16/16
short conception interval: 6 weeks after abortion		+			+			24 4	29.7	2/5
impaired reproductive faculty; conception just following lactation					+			26.1	27.7	4/5
failure during practice of C.R.M.* at the end of reproductive period	+				+	+		42.4	45.6	8/8
irregular cycle after 'insuline fattening cure'; R/duphaston ®: 2 tabl. dd ; coitus condomatus.				+	+			34.9	33.7	5/5
long unintended conception interval (4½ yr.)			+		+			39.0	43.5	9/11
failure during practice of C.R.M.* and irregular menstrual cycle.						+	+	32.5	36.4	5/5

failures during C.R.M.*: i.e. calendar rhythmic method	6×	Average.	
conceptions at the end of reproductive period (>40 years)	2×		
short conception interval	2×	34.0	36.0	5.6/6.2
long unintended conception interval	1×		
endocrinological disturbances: hypothyroidy	1×	Range	
after insuline-cure	1×		
during pharmacological treatment: reserpine	2× (?)	24.4–	27.7–
'spring' and 'autumn' conceptions	12×	42.11	49.9

Table II

Number of patient	Number of registration	Date of birth	Criterion of selection	Phenotype	Karyotype	Sex-chromatin	Complications of pregnancy
1	1471	17–9–'65	KLIPPEL-FEIL and PTERYGIUM COLLI	♀	46,XX	pos	low backpain (ischias)
2	320	8–8–'50	KLIPPEL-FEIL and PTERYGIUM COLLI	♀	46 XX	pos.	low backpain from 3rd till 7th month
3	897	3–8–'58	KLIPPEL-FEIL and PTERYGIUM COLLI	♀	46,XX	pos.	3rd month hospitalised during 7 days for rheuma.
4	1337	7–5–'64	KLIPPEL-FEIL and PTERYGIUM COLLI	♀	46,XX	pos	
5	1026	13–1–'63	KLIPPEL-FEIL and PTERYGIUM COLLI	♀	46,XX	pos.	5th month: blood flow (5 days at rest). hydramnios (at the end of pregnancy)
6	779	30–6–'56	KLIPPEL-FEIL and PTERYGIUM COLLI	♀	47,XXG	pos	till 3rd month drugs against hypertension; 6th month viral infection (10 days at rest)
7	511	25–2–'57	MALE TURNER SYNDROME	♂	46,XY	neg.	decreased child movements
8	1232	14–3–'62	MALE TURNER SYNDROME	♂	46,XY	neg	1st month blood flow; many complaints abdominal pain; increased child movements
9	1523	4–6–'62	MALE TURNER SYNDROME	♂	46,XY	neg.	very few child movements; hydramnios; hyperemesis.
10	629	17–3–'56	NON FAMILIAL MOBIUS SYNDROME	♂	46,XY	neg	
11	1065	8–9–'58	NON FAMILIAL MOBIUS SYNDROME	♀	46,XX	pos	oligohydramnios; hyperemesis; increased child movements
12	1176	3–4–'62	NON FAMILIAL MOBIUS SYNDROME	♀	46,XXqi	pos.	
13	1270	3–3–'66	DECREASE OF SEX-CHROMATIN	♀	45,X/46,XXq+	neg./pos.	6th month: pyelitis
14	172	16–4–'45	ABSENCE OF SEX-CHROMATIN	♀	45,X	neg.	decreased child movements.
15	1228	3–2–'61	ABSENCE OF SEX-CHROMATIN	♀	45,X	neg.	

abdominal or low backpain complaints	3×
polyhydramnios	2×
oligohydramnios	1×
bloodflow	2×
decreased childmovements	3×
increased childmovements	2×
hyperemesis	2×

Complications of parturition		Birth weight	Complications of neonatal period
à terme; haemorrhage just before parturition; protracted progress.		3.300 gr.	cyanosis; dyspnoe; enormous pterygium colli; hospitalised during two months
à terme; difficult and protracted course		±2.500 gr.	cyanosis
1 week overdue; protracted course		3.500 gr.	cried for the first time after 10 minutes
à terme; protracted course		3.140 gr.	cried not spontaneously; somewhat cyanotic
14 days before time; breech presentation; difficult parturition		2.250 gr.	cried only after 10 minutes
6 weeks overdue; protracted course		3.500 gr.	cyanosis, cried after some ticks
during last month continuous contractions; à terme 8 injections of piton		±3.000 gr.	crying very feeble; hypogenitalism; omphalocele; hospitalised during 1 month
		±3.500 gr.	cyanotic and lax, enormous pterygium colli and cutis laxa on abdomen and neck
4 weeks before time: 8 à 10 lt. amniotic fluid containing meconium, placenta accreta		3.300 gr.	cyanotic; groaning very feeble; low body temp.; oedema on hands and feet; hospitalised during 3 months; congenital myeloid reaction
à terme, spontaneous, but too slowly; R/3 injections		±3.500 gr.	cyanotic and very lax
4 weeks before time: breech presentation; amniotic fluid containing meconium		±2.000 gr.	great difficulties of nourishment; 3 months in incubator
		±3.500 gr.	low body temperature
during last 6 weeks continuous contractions; ± 2 weeks overdue		2.700 gr.	crying very feeble; a little cyanotic; low body temperature; hospitalised during 4 weeks
à terme; breech presentation		±2.000 gr.	refused breastfeeding
		3.000 gr.	
overdue	3×	±2.980 gr.	cyanosis 7×
before time	3×		dyspnoea 1×
protracted course	7×		low body temperature 3×
breech presentation	3×		lymphoedema 1×
placenta accreta	1×		
ante partum haemorrhage	1×		
amniotic fluid containing meconium	2×		

Table III

Number of patient	Number of registration	Date of birth	Criterion of selection	Phenotype	Karyotype	Sex-chromatin	Small stature ≤ 3rd perc.	Retarded skeletal age	Microbrachycephaly	Low posterior hairline	Short neck	Webbed neck	Low set ears	Malformed ears	Hearing impairment	Ptosis eyelid	Strabismus	Others
1	1471	17–9–'65	KLIPPEL-FEIL and PTERYGIUM COLLI	♀	46,XX	pos.	+	—	—	+	+	+	+		+	+	—	+
2	320	8–8–'50	KLIPPEL-FEIL and PTERYGIUM COLLI	♀	46,XX	pos.	+		+	+	+	+	+			+		
3	897	3–8–'58	KLIPPEL-FEIL and PTERYGIUM COLLI	♀	46,XX	pos.	+		—	+	+	+	+		+	+	+	+
4	1337	7–5–'64	KLIPPEL-FEIL and PTERYGIUM COLLI	♀	46,XX	pos.	+	+	+	+	+	+	+	+	+	+	+	+
5	1026	13–1–'63	KLIPPEL-FEIL and PTERYGIUM COLLI	♀	46,XX	pos.	+	—	—	+	+	+	+	+	+	+	+	+
6	779	30–6–'56	KLIPPEL-FEIL and PTERYGIUM COLLI	♀	47,XXG	pos.	+ .	—	+	+	+	+				+		
7	511	25–2–'57	MALE TURNER SYNDROME	♂	46,XY	neg.	+	+	+	+	+	+	+	+	+	+		
8	1232	14–3–'62	MALE TURNER SYNDROME	♂	46,XY	neg.	>10°p.		+	+	—	+	+		—	—		+
9	1523	4–6–'62	MALE TURNER SYNDROME	♂	46,XY	neg.	+	+	+	+	+	+	+		+	+	+	
10	629	17–3–'56	NON FAMILIAL MÖBIUS SYNDROME	♂	46,XY	neg.	>25°p.	—	—	+	—	—	+			+	+	+
11	1065	8–9–'58	NON FAMILIAL MÖBIUS SYNDROME	♀	46,XX	pos.	+	—	+		—	—			—	+	+	+
12	1176	3–4–'62	NON FAMILIAL MÖBIUS SYNDROME	♀	46,XXqi	pos.	>25°p.	+	+		—	—	+	+	+	+	+	+
13	1270	3–3–'66	DECREASE OF SEX-CHROMATIN	♀	45,X/46,XXq+	neg./pos.	+		—		—	—			—		+	
14	172	16–4–'45	ABSENCE OF SEX-CHROMATIN	♀	45,X	neg.	+		+		+	—				+	—	
15	1228	3–2–'61	ABSENCE OF SEX-CHROMATIN	♀	45,X	neg.	>10°p.		+		—	—	—		—		+	

Narrow arched palate	Kyphosis	Scoliosis	Cubitus valgus	Span > stature	Nuchal ribs	Thoracic anomalies	Muscle defects	Kryptorchism	Further dysplasias and other pathology	Psychometric evaluation
+	+	+	+	—		+	+	o	herniation of cerebral tissue through the foramen magnum; cervical vertebrae	low grade imbecile
			+	+	+		+	o	bilateral subluxation of the hips; anovulatory irregular cycles	medium grade idiot
	+		+	+		+		o	congenital anomaly of the system of middle ear ossicles — latent diabetes (disturbed G.T.C.)	borderline
+	+		+	+		+		o	widened lateral ventricles	low grade imbecile
	+	+	—			+		o	Goldenhar's syndrome (dermoid of limbus corneae and auricular appendages)	medium grade feeble-minded
+	+		—	+	+	+		o	Down's phenotype	low grade idiot
	+	+	+	—		+		+	omphalocele; acrocyanosis and temporary steatorrhoea	medium grade imbecile
+			—	+	+			+	extra posterior cervical skin; 3rd ventricle widened	medium grade imbecile
+			+	+		+		+	congenital heart disease	low up to medium grade imbecile
	+		+		+		+	—	widened lateral ventricles; polythely; acrocyanosis; increased gonadotrophines and hypogenitalism; osteoporosis	low grade imbecile
+			+					o	latent diabetes (disturbed G.T.C.)	low grade imbecile
	+		—	+	+			o	widened lateral ventricles	medium grade imbecile
			+	—				o	small widening of lateral ventricles	low up to medium grade imbecile
+	+	+	+		+			o	primary amenorrhea; osteoporosis	high grade idiot
+	+		+	—		+		o	nephrotic syndrome accompanied with persistant diarrhoea, improved after prednison treatment	medium grade imbecile

2. The concept of overripeness ovopathy implies a pleiotropic teratogenic factor and might explain the highly variable symptomatology in the above mentioned patients.

It is wellknown that none of the Turner stigmata can be called pathognomonic for the s.T. Short stature is the rule but can be absent. In two of the patients with monosomy for the short arm of X (nos. 12 and 15) height exceeds the 25th and the 10th percentile respectively. This is difficult to reconcile with the hypothesis of FERGUSON-SMITH (1965) (JONGBLOET 1971b).

The varying degrees of mental retardation present in this series of patients are not surprising, though it should be noted that persons with Turner's and allied syndromes can be of normal and even superior intelligence. Abnormal encephalogrammes, irregular test profiles and widely different forms of mental disturbance were encountered in s.T., irrespective of the karyogramme (MONEY and GRANOFF 1965). Statistically there exists no correlation between the above and the presence or absence of sex chromatin, or, in cases of mosaicism, the ratio of abnormal to normal cell clones (ZÜBLIN 1969). From the view-point of overripeness ovopathy they all might be traced back to concomitant developmental cerebral anomalies. The same holds true for co-existing malformations of the cranial base, of heart and kidneys, of the umbilicus, etc.

ANDERSON et al. (1969) demonstrated that 32% of s.T. patients showed a conductive or mixed type of hearing impairment. Cephalometric analysis proved the external auditory canals to be caudally displaced, which is in agreement with the clinical observation of low-set ears. Moreover, mild perception deafness was found in 64%. Hearing impairment in our patients with Klippel-Feil's, non-familial Möbius', and male Turner's syndromes might therefore not come unexpectedly, if our assumption that they have a common cause, i.e. overripeness ovopathy, is true.

The neonatal myeloid reaction in a patient with male Turner's syndrome (no. 9) and the latent juvenile diabetes in patients no. 3 (with brevicollis congenita) and no. 11 (with Möbius' syndrome) seem to be clinical enigmata. However, they too, become more understandable if one accepts that these syndromes might be the result of overripeness ovopathy.

The relatively frequent occurrence of leukaemia and leukaemoid reaction in neonatal life in children with trisomy 21 is common knowledge. It is less known that it has also been described in s.T., in trisomy D., in congenital heart disease, in Klippel-Feil anomaly, Poland's syndrome, and st. B.U. (MILLER et al. 1969, BOAZ et al. 1971). WERTELECKI et al. (1970) showed a preponderance of neurogenic tumors too, in s.T. and suggested that this tendency may be shared by 'syndromes with a Turner phenotype irrespective of a visible chromosomal defect'.

On the other hand, diabetes mellitus, associated with brevicollis congenita or with Möbius' syndrome, seems to be rare. However, diabetes not only occurs significantly more frequently in patients with s.T. (NIELSEN et al. 1969), and in the syndromes of Down and Klinefelter, but also in children with other malformations (BARTÁ et al. 1968). The latter authors therefore advanced the opinion that damage to germ cells might be the primary cause of such combinations. Overripeness ovopathy offers a suitable base for this line of thought.

3. The concept of overripeness ovopathy might be of assistance in distinguishing between the syndromes of the B.U.T. spectrum and those of a genetic origin.

Möbius' syndrome is known to occur in familial as well as in nonfamilial forms. If the former are inherited and the latter might be due to overripeness ovopathy, this offers a means to distinguish between them. In that case namely, the former are to be considered genocopies and will follow mendelian rules. The same holds true for 'pure' gonadal dysgenesis, testicular feminization (Morris' syndrome) and familial male pseudohermaphroditism, which can be categorized as genocopies. The non-familial forms of Möbius' syndrome on the other hand, and many allied conditions brought under notice, can be traced by using the set of diagnostic criteria for overripeness ovopathy developed elsewhere (JONGBLOET 1971d).

Two problems still have to be faced since ostensibly they are not in keeping with overripeness ovopathy as a possible aetiology of s.T.: firstly, the lack of age-effect in the mother and, secondly, the possibility of familial occurrence of the Turner phenotype. Some authors are of the opinion that elderly expectant women do not run an increased risk of bearing a child with complete or partial absence of an X chromosome, or with structural deficiencies of that chromosome (LINDSTEN 1963, VAN DEN BERGHE 1966, COURT-BROWN et al. 1969). However, PENROSE (1961), noted a 'bimodal tendency' in the maternal age curve, and POLANI (1962) a 'small tail of advanced maternal ages'. In our four patients with gonosomal aberrations (nos. 12, 13, 14, 15) the maternal age at birth, too, was rather advanced, resp. 42; 4, 34; 8, 39; 0 and 32; 5 years. Obviously, our data do not allow to draw any conclusions. In any case, even if there exists a modest age-effect in s.T., it strongly contrasts with the pronounced age-effect in Down's and Klinefelter's syndromes. The problem then arises how to explain this difference in age-effect. It should be recalled that these three syndromes seem to follow the same seasonal trend in their respective birth curves, which led us to suggest overripeness ovopathy as a possible common aetiology (JONGBLOET 1971a). Now the average maternal age at which spontaneous abortions occur seems to be the same for normal embryos and for those with a 45, X configuration (BOUÉ and BOUÉ 1970). In other words, there are no indications that the lack of age-effect in s.T. is the result of a preferential age-effect in pregnancy wastage of 45, X embryos. If allowed to speculate, we should like to venture the following hypothesis: In both Down's and Klinefelter's syndromes a combination of both maternal and paternal age-effects is operative, while in s.T. paternal contribution is somehow lacking. If such might be the case, the average maternal age at delivery would be linked exclusively to the fertile period of the female, which on average is shorter than that of the male. In the absence of a paternal age-effect, abnormalities resulting from premenopausal conceptions might be balanced by those from high-risk conception groups at the beginning of the fertile period. The result then would be that the *average* maternal age at the birth of a child with s.T. would not differ greatly from that at the birth of a normal one. As a matter of fact indeed, some authors observed an increased frequency of s.T. in children of primiparae and adolescent girls (LENZ 1959, BOYER et al. 1961, VAN DEN BERGHE 1966).

A second reason to hesitate before accepting overripeness ovopathy as a cause of Turner phenotype and karyotype might be the occurrence of familial cases suggesting hereditary mechanisms. JOSSO et al. (1963) and BOCZKOWSKI et al. (1969) described the occurrence of more than one case of s.T. in one family. The latter suggested several possibilities: (1) it might be coincidence, (2) it might be a suggestion of a transmitted familial character and (3) it might indicate a familial tendency for loss at anaphase or non-disjunction during meiosis. The last possibility was considered to be the most probable one, on account of a number of reports concerning various chromosomal aberrations in one sibship. On the other hand, maternal factors such as endocrinological disturbances and 'marginal' damage of the ovaries might predispose to pathological conceptions, a.o. to twin pregnancies, chromosomal aberrations, abortions and births of children with congenital malformations (JONGBLOET 1971a and d). Several investigators, indeed, found an increase in twin pregnancies in the sibships of 45, X patients (LINDSTEN 1963, NANCE and UCHIDA 1964, VAN DEN BERGHE 1966, NIELSEN 1968). In our own study we, too, observed a high frequency of presumably spontaneous abortions (22.8%), still-births (4.8%), congenital aberrations (9.5%) and multiple births (6.5%). These data were calculated after subtraction of the propositi.

Finally, a few remarks should be made concerning the so-called syndrome of Noonan. In 1965 SUMMITT et al. separated a group of patients characterized by congenital heart disease, Turner stigmata and a *normal* karyotype (both XX and XY) as a distinct nosological entity from the B.U.T. spectrum, one of the reasons being that some of these patients were found to cluster in certain sibships. These authors therefore suggested that the syndrome be called the 'Noonan syndrome' after Dr. Jacqueline NOONAN, who was the first to call attention to this combination of symptoms. Because of the occurrence in sibships, they spoke of a 'genocopy of s.T.'. Though the first impression was that this was indeed a hereditary syndrome, demonstration of the exact mode of transmission met with many difficulties. One of these was that it appeared to be transmitted exclusively through the mother, and that, on closer inspection, the mother herself sometimes showed Turner stigmata or 'minor manifestations' (POLANI et al. 1967, NORA and SINHA 1969, JACKSON and LEFRAK 1969). The difficulties encountered have given rise to quite a number of possible explanations. Submicroscopic chromosomal aberrations, hidden mosaicism or multifactorial inheritance were suggested by KAPLAN et al. (1968), autosomal recessive inheritance by ABDEL-SALAM and TEMTAMY (1969), polygenic mode of inheritance by SUMMITT (1969), X-linked dominant inheritance by POLANI et al. (1967) and by NORA and SINHA (1969) and finally autosomal dominant transmission with variable expression by LEVY et al. (1970).

Returning to the observation of mothers with Turner stigmata giving birth to children with the syndrome described, this could also be interpreted as follows: A woman, herself showing the signature of (mild) overripeness ovopathy, ('marginal affections', JONGBLOET 1971a, b and d) and thereby constitutionally predisposed to abnormal conceptions, is apt to produce children with congenital aberrations, tending to cluster in the family and, consequently, mimicking genetic transmission patterns. For this reason we are inclined to view Noonan's syndrome as one of the many consequences of overripeness ovopathy, and not as a genocopy of s.T.

SUMMARY

In this study 6 patients with Klippel-Feil anomaly and dystrophia brevicolli congenita (Nielsen), 3 patients with male Turner syndrome, 3 patients with non-familial Möbius' syndrome and finally 3 females with a decreased amount or absence of sex chromatin are discussed. In 13 out of 15 of these patients a situation was shown to have been present at conception which could have led to overripeness of the egg. A unifying concept of overripeness ovopathy as aetiology appears to offer an explanation for both the pluriformity of the symptomatology and the overlapping within the complex of syndromes which can be included in the Bonnevie-Ullrich-Turner spectrum. Furthermore, this concept might explain why the above mentioned syndromes do not follow genetic rules as do their genocopies, such as the familial Möbius' syndrome, 'pure' gonadal dysgenesis, testicular feminization and familial male pseudo-hermaphroditism. The age-effect seems to be absent in Turner's, in contrast to Down's and Klinefelter's syndromes. Admittedly, this is difficult to reconcile with the concept of overripeness ovopathy. The sometimes observed phenomenon of clustering of Turner's pheno- and karyotypes within certain sibships might be explained by assuming a constitutional maternal factor, predisposing to pathological conceptions. This factor might itself be due to overripeness ovopathy. Finally, present concepts concerning 'Noonan's syndrome' are discussed.

ACKNOWLEDGEMENTS

We are grateful for critical remarks by and fruitful discussions with Dr. T. D. Stahlie, Professor of paediatrics, Free University of Amsterdam, and with Dr. P. J. Waardenburg, former Lecturer in Medical Genetics, Oosterbeek, The Netherlands. The cytogenetic examinations were carried out in the cytogenetic laboratory under Dr. Ca. van Kempen, the metabolic examinations in the biochemical laboratory under Dr. S. Lormans-Lauwers, the roentgenologic examinations in the X-ray department under Dr. F. Peeters. The genealogical research was done by drs. G. M. A. Jongbloet-van Houtte, historian, and the audiologic examinations by L. Verbeeck. The psychological evaluation of the patients was performed by Drs. J. van Deursen, Drs. P. Engels and Drs. H. Gresnigt, psychologists, all of them staff members of Huize 'Maria Roepaan'.

The Tables were drawn by Miss A.M.A. Verstraaten and Drs. J. H. M. Berden and the translation was carried out by Dr. J. A. M. and Mrs. G. A. van der Mey, B.Sc. We thank them cordially for their cooperation.

REFERENCES

ABDEL-SALAM, E. and S. A. TEMTAMY, Familial Turner phenotype. *J. Pediat.* 74: 67, 1969.

ANDERSON, H., R. FILIPSSON, E. FLUUR, B. KOCH, J. LINDSTEN and E. WEDENBERG, Hearing impairment in Turner's syndrome. *Acta oto-laryng.* Suppl. 247: 26 pp., 1969.

BARTÁ, L., M. SELLYEI and K. SCHMIDT, Uber die Varianten des Turner Syndroms. *Acta paediat. Acad. Sci. hung.* 9: 305, 1968.

BERGHE, H. VAN DEN, *Het zogenaamde syndroom van Turner.* Standaard Wetenschappelijke uitgeverij, Antwerpen, 1966.

BOAZ, D., J. W. MACE and R. W. GOTLIN, Poland's syndrome and leukaemia. *Lancet* i: 349, 1971.

BOCZKOWSKI, K., E. HERMAN and M. JEDRZEJEWSKI, The presence of Turner's syndrome with 45, X karyotype in two generations. *Amer. J. Obstet. Gynec.* 103: 597, 1969.

BOUÉ, J. G. and A. BOUÉ, Les aberrations chromosomiques dans les avortements spontanés humains. *Presse méd.* 78: 635, 1970.

BOYER, S. H., M. A. FERGUSON SMITH and M. M. GRUMBACH, The lack of influence of parental age and birth order in the aetiology of nuclear sex chromatin-negative Turner's syndrome. *Amer. J. hum. Genet.* (Lond.) 25: 215, 1961.

CAFLISCH, A., *Das Pterygium und sein Vorkommen bei verschiedenen Zuständen multipler Abartungen.* (Status Bonnevie-Ullrich, Dystrophia brevicolli congenita, Turner-Syndrom, Arthromyodysplasia congenita). Leemann A. G., Zürich, 1952.

COTTERMAN, C. W. and H. F. FALLS, Unilateral developmental anomalies in sisters (Status Bonnevie-Ullrich). *Amer. J. hum. Genet.* 1: 203, 1949.

COURT BROWN, W. M., P. LAW and P. G. SMITH, Sex-chromosome aneuploidy and parental age. *Ann. hum. Genet.* 33: 1, 1969.

DANIS, P., Sur les anomalies congénitales de la totalité oculaire d'origine musculaire et en particulier sur le syndrome de Stilling–Turk–Duane. *Ann. Oculist.* 181: 148, 1948.

FERGUSON SMITH, M. A., Karyotype-phenotype correlations in gonadal dysgenesis and their bearing on the pathogenesis of malformations. *J. med. Genet.* 2: 142, 1965.

FLAVELL, G., Webbing of the neck with Turner's syndrome in male. *Brit. J. Surg.* 31: 150, 1943.

GOLDENHAR, M., Associations des malformations de l'oeil et de l'oreille en particulier le syndrome dermoïde épibulbaire–appendices auriculaires–fistula auris congenita et ses relations avec la dysostose mandibulo-faciale. *J. Génét. hum.* 1: 243, 1952.

GORDON, H., A case of Poland's Syndrome: congenital unilateral brachy-syndactyly with partial absence of the Pectoralis major muscle. *S. Afr. med. J.* 44: 285, 1970.

JONGBLOET, P. H., Overripeness of the egg. *Maandschr. Kindergeneesk.* 36: 352, 1968.

JONGBLOET, P. H., The intriguing phenomenon of gametopathy and its disastrous effects on the human progeny. *Ibidem* 37: 261, 1969.

JONGBLOET, P. H., An investigation into the occurrence of overripeness ovopathy in the normal population. *Ibidem* 38: 228, 1970.

JONGBLOET, P. H., Chromosomal aberrations and month of birth. *Lancet* ii: 1317, 1970

JONGBLOET, P. H., Month of birth and gametopathy. *Clin. Genet.* 2: issue 5, nov. 1971 (a).

JONGBLOET, P. H., Status Bonnevie-Ullrich and Turner's syndrome. Overripeness ovopathy as a unifying concept. Part I. (in the press) 1971 (b).

JONGBLOET, P. H., Diagnostic criteria for overripeness ovopathy. *Maandschr. Kindergeneesk.* 39: 251, 1971 (d).

JOSSO, N., J. DE GROUCHY, J. FRÉZAL and M. LAMY, Le syndrome de Turner familial. Etude de deux familles avec caryotypes XO et XX. *Ann. Pédiat.* 10: 163, 1963.

KÄLLEN, B. and J. WINBERG, A Swedish register of congenital malformations. *Pediatrics* 41: 765, 1968.

KAPLAN, M. S., J. R. OPITZ and F. R. GOSSET, Noonan's syndrome. *Amer. J. Dis. Child.* 116: 359, 1968.

LENZ, W., Der Einfluss des Alters der Eltern und der Geburtennummer auf angeborene patholo-gische Zustände beim Kind. II. *Acta genet.* 9: 249, 1959.

LINDSTEN, J., *The nature and origin of X-chromosome aberrations in Turner's syndrome.* Almqvist & Wiksell, Stockholm, 1963.

MCKUSICK, V. A., On lumpers and splitters, or the nosology of genetic disease. *Birth Defects: Orig. Art. Ser.* 5: 23, 1969.

MIETTINEN, O. S., M. L. REINER and A. S. NADAS, Seasonal incidence of coarctation of the aorta. *Brit. Heart J.* 32: 103, 1970.

MILLER, R. W., Childhood cancer and congenital defects. A study of US. death certificates during the period 1960–1966. *Pediat. Res.* 3: 389, 1969.

MONEY, J. and D. GRANOFF, IQ and the somatic stigmata of Turner's syndrome. *Amer. J. ment. defic.* 70: 69, 1965.

NANCE, W. E. and I. UCHIDA, Turner's syndrome, twinning and an unusual variant of G.-6-P.D. *Amer. J. hum. Genet.* 16: 380, 1964.

NIELSEN, H., Congenital dystrophia of the neck (Klippel-Feil Syndrome). *Hospitalstidende* 409: 77, 1934.

NIELSEN, J., Twins and Klinefelter's syndrome. *A. Ge. Me. Ge.* 17: 385, 1968.

NIELSEN, J., K. JOHANSEN and H. YDE, The frequency of diabetes mellitus in patients with Turner's syndrome and pure gonadal dysgenesis. Blood glucose plasma insulin and growth hormone level during an oral glucose tolerance test. *Acta endocr.* 62: 251, 1969.

NOONAN, J. A. and D. A. EHMKE, Associated noncardiac malformations in children with congenital heart disease. *J. Pediat.* 63: 468, 1963.

NORA, J. J. and A. SINHA, Inheritance of the Turner phenotype. *Birth Defects: Orig. Art. Ser.* 5: 29, 1969.

PENROSE, L. S., Parental age and non-disjunction. In: *Human chromosomal abnormalities*. Davidson W. M. and D. R. Smith ed., London, p. 116, 1961.

POLANI, P. E., Sex chromosome anomalies in man. In: *Chromosomes in Medicine*. Hamerton J. L. ed., London, p. 73, 1962.

POLANI, P. E., R. ANGELL and N. POLANI, Ullrich's syndrome. *Lancet* ii: 421, 1967.

SUMMITT, R. L., J. M. OPITZ and D. W. SMITH, Noonan's syndrome in the male. *J. Pediat.* 67: 936, 1965.

SUMMITT, R. L., Turner syndrome and Noonan's syndrome. *J. Pediat.* 74: 155, 1969.

ULLRICH, O., Uber typische Kombinationsbilder multipler Abartungen. *Z. Kinderheilk.* 49: 271, 1930.

WERTELECKI, W., J. F. FRAUMENI and J. J. MULVIHILL, Nongonadal neoplasia in Turner's syndrome. *Cancer* 26: 486. 1970.

ZÜBLIN, W., *Chromosomale Aberrationen und Psyche*. S. Karger, Basel-New York, p. 42–61, 1969.

CHAPTER VII

DIAGNOSTIC CRITERIA FOR OVERRIPENESS OVOPATHY

BY

P. H. JONGBLOET*

INTRODUCTION

Infectious diseases and endocrinological disturbances in the mother during pregnancy have long been considered as a cause of Down's syndrome. However, in 1922 already HALBERTSMA had collected fourteen presumably dizygotic pairs of twins of which one child was healthy and the other suffering from Down's syndrome. From this observation he concluded that the cause of Down's syndrome was not peristatic, but was to be found in an abnormal egg cell, *i.e.* in a 'vitium primae formationis'. Later on, GEYER (1941) spoke of a 'dysplasmatic ovum' and LANDE-CHAMPAIN (1954) of a 'border-line ovum'. The latter was 'unable to find any maternal illnesses or accidents', investigating the first months of pregnancy of 150 mothers of patients with Down's syndrome. But she was struck by the 'highly revealing circumstances in a great many cases just before or at the time of conception'. As such she mentioned physiological exhaustion of the ovaries around the menopause, as well as temporary, primary or secondary, dysfunction of the ovaries, due to thyroid gland deficiency, acute and sub-chronic diseases, short intervals between pregnancies, local disturbances in ovaries and tubae, and finally psychiatric disorders around the conception. On the other hand, WAARDENBURG already suspected in 1932, and others after him, that the syndrome was caused by a chromosomal aberration, which was confirmed by LEJEUNE's discovery of an extra G chromosome in the cells of these patients (1959). Therewith the controversy between supporters and opponents of the 'germinal' theory seemed definitively settled.

The drawback of this discovery was that malformations with chromosomal aberrations became separated from those with normal chromosomes. Thus the relationship between mongolism and congenital malformations such as

---

* Paediatrician, medical director Huize 'Maria Roepaan', Observation and Treatment Centre of mentally retarded, Ottersum (L), The Netherlands.

Maandschr. Kindergeneesk., 39 : 251; 1971.

cebocephaly, cyclopy, anencephaly etc., recognized by VAN DER SCHEER (1919), HALBERTSMA (1922) and many others, was lost sight of. However, the notion of this relationship seems to be still of importance. For, it might lead to the recognition of teratologic factors causing both the syndromes now known to show chromosomal aberrations and those without these.

Such a common cause might be overripeness of the egg (JONGBLOET 1968, 1969, 1970 and 1971a, b and c). This concept is derived from experimental animal investigations (*e.g.* PFLÜGER 1882, WITSCHI 1952, MIKAMO 1968), and provides a biological explanation for congenital anomalies with and without chromosomal aberrations in man. We were able to show, first in parents of mentally retarded children and later also in an aselect population, that there are evident relations between a 'positive overripeness anamnesis' and abnormal progeny. This might imply that, by and large, factors influencing the germ cells are perhaps more important than those operating at a later stage in the development of the embryo, *i.e.* the peristatic factors.

On the other hand, many abnormalities formerly thought to be of genetic origin might, on closer examination, also found to be caused by overripeness ovopathy. Evidently, the increase of such abnormalities in lower socioeconomic classes, in primogeniture, in premenopausal reproduction or in other categories influenced by circumstantial factors, are arguments against a genetic origin. As a matter of fact, arguments commonly used heretofore *against* a genetic origin of certain specified abnormalities can, by the same token, be used *in favour* of overripeness ovopathy.

When the above-mentioned causes of congenital aberrations are arranged chronologically according to their time of operation, the sequence must be (1) genetic, (2) germinal and (3) peristatic factors. The criteria for the first are that mostly they can be traced back to former generations. Damage to the germ cells by definition occurs just before or around fertilization, while peristatic damage takes place during pregnancy. Overripeness ovopathy has to be assigned to the group of germinal causes, that is to say it occupies a central position, while on the one hand its effects can be mimicked by genetic factors (genocopies), on the other they can be copied by peristatic factors (phenocopies) (cf. Table 1.).

TABLE 1.

endogenous	exogenous	
genetic factors	germinal factors	peristatic factors
located in the DNA of the chromosomes (possibly also in the cytoplasm) DNA mutation	causing abnormalities of nucleus and cytoplasm of egg and sperm	causing abnormal organogenesis in embryo (embryopathy) and in foetus (foetopathy)
genocopy	overripeness ovopathy	phenocopy

Such a distinction is of real importance, not only from the viewpoint of nosological categorization, but also for genetic counselling and eventually for prevention. Therefore, it is important to elucidate the criteria, by which deviations caused by intrafollicular and/or intratubal overripeness, can be recognized, in order to enable one to distinguish between geno- and phenocopies. These criteria still have to be deduced empirically on the one hand from experimental animal research and on the other from knowledge of analogous phenomena in human pathology, *i.e.* in those situations in which circumstantial evidence exists for ageing of the egg cell.

It is the purpose of this article to formulate the diagnostic criteria which a malformation or any other disease has to answer, to make overripeness ovopathy acceptable as aetiology. After some theoretical considerations concerning each criterion, attention will be paid to data from the literature, which will be checked with our criteria in as far as they are related to Down's syndrome, dysplasias of the central nervous system, palatocheiloschizis and congenital hip disease. Then the same approach will be made for less familiar and little investigated developmental malformations, such as congenital thyroid dysplasia and DiGeorge's syndrome. The names of the authors, who have reported supporting arguments, will be collected in the tables 2, 3, 4 and 5. (table 2: criterion I to V; table 3: criterion VI: table 4: criterion VII and table 5: criterion VIII).

CRITERION I: MALFORMATIONS CAUSED BY OVERRIPENESS OVOPATHY DO NOT OR ONLY VERY RARELY OCCUR FAMILIALLY

Since overripeness of the egg cell is caused by exogenous factors, that is factors outside the egg, it is to be expected that the resulting aberrations will only rarely occur more than once in the same family and, consequently, will not follow classical genetic laws.

Malformations occurring frequently, such as Down's syndrome, can however mimic genetic inheritance. Consequently, a genetic cause was never completely rejected and in about 3% of all cases one can detect a translocation-chromosome or an extra G chromosome in a mosaic parent. In these peculiar cases the cause of the chromosomal aberration can indeed be traced back to a former generation. Also, malformations of the C.N.S., especially because of their high prevalence, are sometimes thought to be the result of an interaction between 'genetic' and 'environmental' causation (CARTER et al. 1967 and 1969). YEN and MACMAHON (1968), on the other hand, found the 'recurrence risk' of C.N.S. aberrations to be the same for children of the same mother but of a different father (maternal half-siblings) and for children of the same mother and father (full siblings). They considered this observation difficult to reconcile with genetic inheritance and held a 'still unidentified environmental factor' responsible. Also, the lack of consanguineous marriages in the ascendency of patients with these malformations (RECORD and MCKEOWN 1950) argues against (recessive) inheritance as a causal factor. NANCE (1969) attempts to find a compromise in this controversy by considering the same 'maternal recurrence risk' for 'full' and 'half-siblings' reconciliable with 'cytoplasmatic inheritance'. Later on we shall point out the possibility of a constitutional factor in the mother caused by a lability in the hypothalamus-pituitary-ovary system (see criterion VI). This factor then might predispose to pregnancy wastage as well as to various forms of congenital malformations, including the occasional recurrence of a malformation already produced before. Such a constitutional maternal factor provides in our opinion a better explanation for the 'maternal recurrence risk' in 'half-siblings' than 'cytoplasmatic inheritance.'

CRITERION II: MALFORMATIONS CAUSED BY OVERRIPENESS OVOPATHY OBVIOUSLY OCCUR FREQUENTLY IN BOTH MONOZYGOTIC TWINS OF EQUAL SIZE, BUT MORE ESPECIALLY IN THE SMALLER ONE OF SUCH A TWIN PAIR

It was pointed out long ago that monozygotic twinning should be considered an aberration *per se* and that the impetus to this form of twinhood can be the cause of intrauterine mortality and congenital malformations. STOCKARD (1920–1921) concluded from animal experiments that one-egg twins as well as various non-hereditary malformations are due to 'properly timed developmental arrest'. The types and degrees of the malformations exhibited by the smaller component of a twin pair, were exactly similar in kind and degree to the deformities found among single individuals. Therefore STOCKARD considered the double individual with unequal components a most valuable key to an understanding of the cause of malformations. AREY (1923) maintained that these concepts should apply equally well to human abnormalities and twinning, provided the ovum is subject to delay before implantation and to arrest afterwards.

More recent investigators (MORISON 1949, CAMPBELL 1965, NAEYE 1965 and others) believe that discordant malformations in one-egg twins are sometimes caused by vascular anomalies in the double placentation. Anastomosis of vessels ('third circulation') might cause an unequal supply of oxygen and nutrients to the twins (parabiotic syndrome). Here, in our opinion however, cause and effect are not sufficiently distinguished since a disturbance taking place before the placentae are formed might cause both the vascular anomalies and the morphogenetic malformations.

The controversy concerning the origin of discordant one-egg twins, who might have been caused by either exogenous or hereditary factors, mainly centres around the malformations of the C.N.S. (FRÉZAL e.a. 1964, YEN and MacMahon 1968, LAURENCE e.a. 1968, DE BELLEFEUILLE 1969 and NANCE 1969). All these authors agree that these discordancies can hardly be explained on genetic grounds. They consider that other factors, such as environment, must play a part in the aetiology. NANCE (1969), as mentioned before, favours the concept of 'cytoplasmatic inheritance' as a compromise, saying that diversion in monozygotic twins might be due to qualitative and quantitative differences in their share of cytoplasm from the dividing ovum.

Phenotypic variations are also present in the progeny of the armadillo, a South-American mammal, which is known to give birth to monozygotic quadruplets derived from one fertilized egg cell (NEWMAN 1916, STORRS and WILLIAMS 1968). NEWMAN drew attention to the remarkable mirror-image symmetry in these quadruplets. This mirror-image symmetry is sometimes found in human one-egg twins also, both in dermatoglyphs and in body structures. In its extreme form it is encountered in the 'situs inversus' of conjoined twins. This remarkable phenomenon cannot be explained by genetic information alone, or by quantitative differences arising during the division of the cytoplasm, or by vascular anomalies. Presumably it should be seen as a cytoplasmatic disturbance, by which the reorganization of the physiological asymmetry is troubled in one half after cleavage of the fertilized egg or of a blastomere. The factors responsible for this cytoplasmatic disturbance can be looked for outside the ovum at the time of its very first developmental stages.

INGALLS e.a. (1969) and FERM (1969), from experiments with fishes and mammals, conclude that only exogenous factors can be held responsible for conjoined and other monozygotic twins. The frequent occurrence of chromosomal aberrations in one-egg twins, and especially the fact that the members of the twin pair frequently possess a different chromosome pattern (NIELSEN 1967) cannot be understood, unless assuming an exogenous cause. Experiments with eggs of amphibians by WITSCHI (1952) provide an excellent basis for the explanation of discordancy in one-egg twins. After allowing the eggs to become 'overripe', axial duplication was seen to occur, leading to identical twins, sometimes of like, sometimes of different size. In addition, overripe eggs frequently showed deficiencies in the organogenesis and a defective differentiation of various tissues and organ systems.

It is common usage in genetics to compare for a certain malformation, the degree of concordance in one-egg and two-egg twins (SMITH and AASE 1970). It is then assumed that a high degree of concordance in one-egg twins is conclusive evidence of genetic causation. If, however, the stimulus for one-egg twinhood is itself of an exogenous nature, this assumption is not always valid, the more so in case the same exogenous stimulus is known or assumed to induce the malformation concerned.

CRITERION III: MALFORMATIONS CAUSED BY OVERRIPENESS OVOPATHY ARE
OFTEN ACCOMPANIED BY A MULTIPLICITY OF CONGENITAL ANO-
MALIES, INCLUDING 'IDIOPATHIC' MENTAL DEFICIENCY AND
'DEGENERATIVE' STIGMATA

Experimental animal research has shown that overripeness of the egg can lead
to strongly divergent morphological aberrations. Consequently, it is to be
expected that in man these aberrations rarely occur alone but are usually
accompanied by other defects showing a kaleidoscopic variety and changing
expression. So, for instance, disturbances of the C.N.S., palatocheiloschizis and
congenital hip disease are often accompanied by several other congenital
defects (see table 1). In Down's syndrome, too, apart from the typical stigmata,
one may find congenital heart defects, polydactyly, syndactyly, palatoschizis,
harelip, micro- and macrocephaly, malformation of the external ear, spina
bifida, stenoses of the digestive tract, atresia ani, anophthalmia, cataracts, etc.
This implies that quite a few of the malformations encountered from time to
time in combination with Down's syndrome are not linked to the presence
of an extra G chromosome, as is the case with the characteristic features of that
syndrome. These sporadically occurring malformations may be retraced to a
cytoplasmatic disturbance of the egg.

In our opinion many minor defects usually called 'degenerative stigmata' can
be included in this group. Thus SMITH and BOSTIAN (1964) noted in 42% of the
children with 'idiopathic mental retardation' at least three congenital malformations, 80% of which belonged to the group of 'minor defects'. Various
degenerative stigmata and dermatoglyphic aberrations can be explained by
overripeness ovopathy as had been suggested previously (JONGBLOET 1970,
1971a and b). That overripeness of the egg could be operative in influencing
the formation of dermatoglyphic patterns is indicated too by the sometimes
found discordancy of dermatoglyphs of one-egg twins (KARASOVÁ 1969 and
NYLANDER 1970). In this framework the relationship which seems to exist
between various forms of leukaemia and dermatoglyphs (ROSNER 1970) is
intriguing, since MENSER and PURVIS-SMITH (1969) offered the hypothesis
that 'a prenatal teratogen may be responsible for both'.

CRITERION IV: MALFORMATIONS CAUSED BY OVERRIPENESS OVOPATHY ARE
OFTEN ACCOMPANIED BY NON-SPECIFIC CHROMOSOMAL ABER-
RATIONS

Since overripeness of the egg in the experiment can produce both morphological and chromosomal aberrations, it is to be expected that all sorts of
malformations can be found in combination with non-specific chromosomal
aberrations, as well as that they may occur without chromosomal aberrations.

TABLE 2	I Familial occurrence very rare or absent	II In both monozygotic twins of equal size, but more especially only in the small one of such a twin pair	III Accompanied by a multiplicity of other congenital malformations including „idiopathic mental retardation"	IV Accompanied by nonspecific chromosomal aberrations	V Characterized by hypogonadism
Down's syndrome	van der Scheer 1927 Geyer 1941 Oster 1953	Wolff et al. 1962 Nielsen 1967	Oster 1953 Penrose et al. 1966 Ceccarelli et al. 1968 Fabia 1970	Hecht et al. 1969 Chen et al. 1970	Benda 1969 Peters et al. 1969
Anencephaly, meningomyelocoele, spina bifida	Penrose 1957 Frézal et al. 1964 Yen et al. 1968 Horowitz et al. 1969	Yen et al. 1968 de Bellefeuille 1969 Nance 1969 Horowitz 1969	Record et al. 1949 Coffey et al. 1957 Smilkstein 1962 Frézal 1964 Smithells 1965 Erez 1966		Zondek et al. 1965 Bearn 1968
Palatoschizis and palatocheiloschizis	Drillien et al. 1966 Borçbakan 1969 Fraser 1970	Strean 1958 Fraser 1970 Smith et al. 1970 Markovic 1970	Strean 1958 Gilmore et al. 1966 Pannbacker 1968 Gordon 1969 Bardanouve 1969 Fraser 1970	Ingalls 1947 Penrose et al. 1966 Gilmore et al. 1966 Drillien et al. 1966 Ceccarelli et al. 1968	Pannbacker 1968
Congenital hip disease	Nagura 1960 Illyés 1968 Illyés 1969	Illyés 1969 Smith et al. 1970	Record et al. 1958 Nagura 1960 Illyés 1969	Kaufmann et al. 1961 Penrose et al. 1966 Ceccarelli et al. 1968	Nagura 1960
Agenesis and dysgenesis of thyroid gland	McGirr et al. 1955	Warkany et al. 1955 Pickering et al. 1958 Greig et al. 1966	Rundle 1971	Williams et al. 1964 Benda 1969 Lormans-Lauwers et al. 1970	
Dysgenesis of thymus and/or parathyroid glands (DiGeorge syndrome)	Rosen 1968		Rosen 1968 Kretschmer et al. 1968 Dodson et al. 1969 Lischner et al. 1969	Kadowaki et al. 1965 Vogel 1968 Githens et al. 1969 Pergament et al. 1970	Vogel 1968 Dodson et al. 1969

TABLE 3

VI Symptomatic for a maternal constitutional factor

	Suboptimal reproductive history of mother					Organic or minor defects in mother (dermatoglyphs etc.)	Decreased fertility or premenopausal age of grandmother at birth of mother	Aberrant birthcurve of mothers
	Irregular cycles	Impaired generative faculty or premature menopause	Increase of abortions and still-births (pregnancy wastage)	Increase of chromosomal and congenital aberrations in sibship	Increase of multiple pregnancies in sibship			
Down's syndrome	Geyer 1941 Benda 1949 Cowie et al. 1968	Geyer 1941 Benda 1949 Oster 1953 Lande-Champain 1954 Drillien 1968	van der Scheer 1927 Geyer 1941 Benda 1949 Smith et al. 1955 Ingalls et al. 1957 Vanhaelst et al. 1969	van der Scheer 1927 Wright 1963 Hecht et al. 1963 Penrose et al. 1966	Lunn 1959 Wright et al. 1963	Turpin et al. 1953 Penrose 1954 Ingalls et al. 1957 Buck et al. 1969 Priest 1969 Zajaczkowska 1969	Greenberg 1963	Jongbloet 1971
Anencephaly, meningomyelocoele, spina bifida		Still 1927	Record et al. 1949 Record et al. 1950 Coffey et al. 1957 McDonald 1958 Smilkstein 1962 Frézal 1964 Smithells 1965 Erez et al. 1966	Record et al. 1950 Coffey et al. 1958 Hamersma 1966 Yen et al. 1968				
Palatoschizis and palato-cheiloschizis	Drillien et al. 1968	Drillien et al. 1966	Drillien et al. 1966 Gilmore et al. 1966 Tolarova 1969 Fraser 1970	Drillien et al. 1966 Meskin et al. 1969			Drillien et al. 1966	
Congenital hip disease		Record et al. 1958 Illyés 1968		Record et al. 1958				
Agenesis and dysgenesis of thyroid gland								
Dysgenesis of thymus and/or parathyroid glands (DiGeorge syndrome)								

By using this criterion more light may be thrown on the high frequency of a.o. the associations between malignant disease including leukaemia, and the syndromes of Down (HOLLAND et al. 1962) and Bonnevie-Ullrich-Turner (WERTELECKI et al. 1970); further, between diabetes mellitus and Down's, Turner's and Klinefelter's syndromes (MILUNSKY 1970) and, finally, between dysgenesis of thyroid and thymus on the one hand and various chromosomal syndromes on the other (WILLIAMS et al. 1964, KADOWAKI et al. 1965, VOGEL 1968, GITHENS et al. 1969, BENDA 1969 and LORMANS-LAUWERS et al. 1970).

CRITERION V: MALFORMATIONS CAUSED BY OVERRIPENESS OVOPATHY ARE OFTEN CHARACTERIZED BY HYPOGONADISM

In animal experiments overripeness ovopathy can result in gonadal dysplasias, in addition to morphological and chromosomal aberrations. It is therefore to be expected that in human pathology the same occurs, well-known examples being Turner's and Klinefelter's syndromes. Also, patients with trisomy 21 (BENDA 1969) and trisomy D (TOEWS and JONES 1968) often show hypogonadism. Moreover, hypogonadism is regularly observed in congenital malformations without chromosomal aberrations as an accompanying phenomenon. So, for instance, ZONDEK and ZONDEK (1965) and BEARN (1968) found hypogonadism and hypogenitalism in anencephalics.

The occurrence of evident hypogonadism in certain congenital malformations, assumed by us to be caused by overripeness ovopathy, obviously implies the possibility of the existence of minimal gonadal deficiencies also. Such 'marginal hypogonadism' might offer an explanation for a constitutional predisposition towards reproductive failures (cf. following criterion).

CRITERION VI: MALFORMATIONS CAUSED BY OVERRIPENESS OVOPATHY ARE OFTEN A SYMPTOM OF A MATERNAL CONSTITUTIONAL DEFICIENCY WHICH MANIFESTS ITSELF IN A SUBOPTIMAL REPRODUCTIVE HISTORY

Conceivably, a constitutional deficiency in the hypothalamus-pituitary-ovary axis might predispose to disturbances in ovulation, resulting in (1) irregular cycles, varying from anovulatory to aluteal cycles, (2) temporarily and chronically impaired generative faculty or premature menopause, (3) increase in abortions and still-births (pregnancy wastage), (4) increase in the number of children with congenital malformations with or without chromosomal aberrations, and (5) increase in the number of twin pregnancies.

As noted before, the recurrence risk for malformations of the C.N.S. is just as great for maternal half-siblings as for full siblings. This phenomenon is difficult to explain by classical mendelian inheritance, but points to a specific maternal factor. MYRIANTHOPOULOS (1969) came to a similar conclusion after investigating 60.000 pregnancies. In 139 families with children of one mother but different fathers, abnormalities such as afebrile convulsions, severe squint, congenital heart disease, mental retardation, clubfoot and polydactyly were encountered in equal frequency in both groups of half-sibs. In addition the frequency of various aberrations in these families was unusually high and the pregnancy wastage in both half-sibships did not differ significantly. All these findings led the author to conclude that congenital malformations and pregnancy wastage depend largely on maternal factors.

Such maternal factors may be of a hereditary or non-hereditary nature. In the latter category might be placed the marginal effects of overripeness ovopathy. There are indications that mothers of children with Down's syndrome themselves may be the victims of an abortive form of overripeness ovopathy (JONGBLOET 1971a). So for instance (see table 3):
– they show a higher than normal frequency of minor defects, especially of dermatoglyphic variations;
– the age of their own mothers at the time they were born, is higher than average;
– the fluctuations in the month of birth of the mothers concerned seem to differ from that of the normal population by a greater amplitude.

Overripeness ovopathy might thus predispose to abnormal pregnancy products in the next generation. This might lead to the clustering of non-hereditary anomalies within certain families, mimicking heredity.

CRITERION VII: MALFORMATIONS, CAUSED BY OVERRIPENESS OVOPATHY, OCCUR RELATIVELY FREQUENTLY WITH 'HIGH RISK' CONCEPTIONS

Fertilization of an egg cell, which has been damaged by ageing before ovulation (intrafollicularly) or in the tube (intratubally) can be expected in quite a number of situations, all of them featuring in 'high risk' conception groups. As such can be mentioned conceptions in:

1. *First pregnancies especially in adolescents and*

2. *Premenopausal women*
From studies concerning the menstrual cycle during the fertile period of the woman, it is well known that irregularities in the cycle just after menarche and just before menopause tend to be much more pronounced than in between these periods. In both periods there also exists at the same time an impaired reproductive capacity (FRANCIS 1970), and an increase in abortions (STILL 1927 and BRUNNER 1941), still-births and congenital aberrations (STILL 1927, HENDRICKS 1955, STEWART et al. 1969, CANZLER et al. 1969). FEDRICK (1970)

concluded concerning anencephaly: 'The older the primipara, the lower the incidence, but the older the multipara the higher the incidence'.

After adolescence there is still a risk connected with primogeniture. In primigravidae one has to take into account, besides the lability of the cycle, also stress factors and the possibility of intratubal overripeness of the egg after a first fertilizing coitus or in irregular prenuptial sexual relationships (JONG-BLOET 1969 and 1970). In addition, it should be noted that in older couples coition frequency decreases, thereby increasing the chance of intratubal overripeness (GERMAN 1968).

3. Conceptions after a short conception interval and conceptions immediately after a period of oral contraception

On previous occasions we have repeatedly pointed out the precarious situation of the egg during the first cycle(s) after birth, abortion or interruption of oral contraception. Studying the progeny resulting from such conceptions brought us to the conclusion that here, too, one is dealing with a 'high risk' group (JONGBLOET 1969 and 1970).

4. Conceptions after a long unintended conception interval

YERUSHALMY et al. (1956) and JAMES (1968) studied the influence of birth interval and concluded that both early and late foetal death and also neonatal mortality rates increased with a birth interval longer than two years. McNEIL et al. (1970) observed that children with severe autism, schizophrenia, neuroses and school adjustment problems were often born after a relatively long pregnancy interval.

A long unintended conception interval might indicate an impaired generative faculty, e.g. on the basis of disturbances in ovulation. The incidence of prolonged post partum amenorrhea and of long pregnancy intervals also tends to increase with advancing age of the mother (SALBER et al. 1966).

Many authors, including DOWN (1909), VAN DER SCHEER (1919), STILL (1927), BEIDLEMAN (1945), BENDA (1949 and 1969) and INGALLS et al. (1957) observed a long birth interval with Down's syndrome. However, later investigators (SMITH and RECORD 1955, MATSUNAGA 1967, SIGLER et al., 1967, COWIE and SLATER 1968 and MARMOL et al., 1969) found no such difference in duration of pregnancy interval compaired with an age-matched and, in some cases, a date-of-birth-matched control group. These control groups often even consisted of mentally defective patients, other than those with Down's syndrome. From the viewpoint of the overripeness theory such control groups might obviously consist of offspring of mothers in whom circumstances around conception were analogous. Moreover, very rarely a difference has been made between 'short' and 'long' birth intervals. If both 'high risk' conception groups are not analysed separately but taken together, the results of such investigations

TABLE 4	VII 'HIGH RISK' CONCEPTION GROUPS					
	1. Adolescent girls and primiparous women	2. Premeno-pausal women	3. Short conc. interval (after birth, abortion or interruption of oral contraception)	4. Long unintended conception-interval	Endocrinological disturbances	
					5. hypo-thyroidism	6. prediabetes and diabetes
Down's syndrome	van der Scheer 1927 Oster 1953 Lande-Champain 1954 Smiths et al. 1955 Smiths et al. 1955 Tonomura 1966	van der Scheer 1927 Ingalls 1947 Benda 1949 Smiths et al. 1955 Ingalls et al. 1957	Lande-Champain 1954	Down 1909 van der Scheer 1927 Still 1927 Beidleman 1945 Benda 1949 Oster 1953 Ingalls et al. 1957	Geyer 1941 Benda 1949 Lande-Champain 1954 Fialkow 1967 Dallaire et al. 1969 Vanhaelst et al. 1969	Vanhaelst et al. 1969 Milunsky 1970 Navarrete et al. 1970
Anencephaly, meningomye-locoele, spina bifida	Record et al. 1949 Frézal et al. 1964 Cassady 1969 Horowitz et al. 1969 Fedrick 1970	Coffey et al. 1957 Horowitz et al. 1969 Fedrick 1970	Christakos et al. 1969	Still 1927		Comerford 1965 Codaccioni et al. 1969 Navarrete et al. 1970
Palatoschizis and palatocheiloschizis	Strean 1956 Strean 1958 Borçbakan 1969	Gordon et al. 1969 Bardanouve 1969			Drillien et al. 1966	Navarrete et al. 1970
Congenital hip disease	Record et al. 1958 Illyés 1968 Woolf et al. 1968	Record et al. 1958 Woolf et al. 1968	Illyés 1968	Record et al. 1958		
Agenesis and dysgenesis of thyroid gland						Klein et al. 1968
Dysgenesis of thymus and/or parathyroid glands (DiGeorge syndrome)						Klein et al. 1968

7. Conceptions during spring and autumn	8. Conceptions during viral epidemics	9. Conceptions during undernourishment and in lower socio-economic strata	10. Failures during calendar rhythmic method	11. Conceptions under emotional stress	12. Conceptions during treatment with drugs (psychopharm., antihypertensiva and barbiturates)
or review see Jongbloet 1971a	Stoller et al. 1965 Stoller et al. 1966	Klebanow 1948 Robinson et al. 1969	Jongbloet 1969	Klebanow 1948 Lande-Champain 1954 Stott 1961	
or review see Jongbloet and Pacilly 1971	Stoller et al. 1965	Coffey et al. 1957 de Groot 1965 Hamersma 1966 Fedrick 1970 MacMahon et al. 1971	Cross 1968	Klebanow 1948	
or review see Jongbloet and Pacilly 1971				Strean et al. 1956 Strean 1958 Drillien et al. 1966	Drillien et al. 1966
or review see Jongbloet and Pacilly 1971				Illyés 1968	
				Klebanow 1948	

evidently cannot be convincing. The same remarks hold for our own investigations (1969 and 1970) and those of RECORD and McKEOWN (1950) concerning pregnancy intervals in children with malformations of the C.N.S. Finally, COWIE and SLATER (1968) did not take abortions and still-births into account in their calculations of pregnancy interval.

5. Conceptions in mothers with thyroid gland disturbances

Hypothyroidism can give rise to barely noticeable disturbances in the menstrual cycle, but also to anovulation and amenorrhea (ROSENBERG 1969, LEPRAT and VALCKE 1969). Therefore it is conceivable that diminished fertility, increase in the rate of abortions, premature births, still-births and congenital malformations with or without chromosomal aberrations in hypothyroid women might again be primarily due to disturbed ovulation. FIALKOW (1967), DALLAIRE (1969) and many others detected thyroid autoantibodies in the plasma in mothers of patients with Down's syndrome. This gave rise to FIALKOW's (1964) hypothesis that auto-immune processes may 'on occasion be responsible for the birth of aneuploid children'. It is not unlikely that thyroid autoantibodies cause hypothyroidism, resulting in cycle disturbances and possibility of intrafollicular overripeness.

6. Conceptions in prediabetic and diabetic mothers

In animals (CHIERI et al. 1969) as well as in man (SANDSTRÖM 1969, VAITUKAITIS and MELBY 1969) relationships are known between ovulation disturbances and dysfunction of pancreas and adrenal cortex. The well-known increase in pregnancy wastage, births of children with congenital aberrations and pregnancy complications in mothers with a decreased glucose tolerance is generally exclusively attributed to peristatic factors. However, a distinction should be made between macrosomy on the one hand, which can be ascribed to a disturbed glucose homeostasis, and pregnancy wastage on the other. The latter, in our opinion, could be the consequence of ovopathy, since the pregnancy wastage is hardly reduced when adequate treatment is started *after* conception. NAVARRETE et al. (1970), on the contrary, observed no signs of pre-eclampsia, polyhydramnios, still-births, oversized babies or infants with congenital malformations in a group of prediabetic women, who had received adequate treatment *before* the beginning of pregnancy.

7. Conceptions in 'spring' and 'autumn'

The remarkable relationship between conceptions in 'spring' and 'autumn' and the increase of pregnancy complications, still-births, congenital deviations with or without chromosomal aberrations, of various forms of psychopathology and mental retardation has been commented on elsewhere (JONGBLOET 1971a).

8. Conceptions during viral epidemics

The controversy concerning increase in number of children with Down's syndrome and other congenital malformations, born nine months after an epidemic of virus hepatitis (STOLLER and COLLMAN 1965 and 1966) or of rubella (ROBINSON et al. 1969) has not ended yet (STARK and RUDZKI 1970). It seems important to draw into this discussion the above mentioned increase of pathological conceptions during definite seasons. It does seem likely that a disturbance in the subtle pattern of ovulation could occur during subclinical or clinical viral infections. The cause then might not be viral ovopathy, as assumed by some authors, but overripeness ovopathy as a consequence of the contact with the virus.

9. Conceptions during malnutrition and in socio-economic lower class families

Connections between deficient nutrition and decreased fertility are well-known in many animals. An analogous connection between malnutrition and cycle disturbances or temporary amenorrhea is also assumed in man (e.g. SOUTHAM 1966). MALKANI and MIRCHANDANI observed in India an inverse correlation between the duration of amenorrhea post partum and income of the head of the family. During World War II ROBINSON (1943) noted a similar tendency in British women from lower economic classes. From these data an increase in disturbances in the ovulatory mechanism, with as a consequence overripeness ovopathy, might be expected in periods of undernourishment.

KLEBANOW (1948) reported an eight-fold increase of children with Down's syndrome as well as a disproportional increase of children with many other malformations among 1430 Jewish women who had become pregnant in the first years after release from a concentration camp. Relationships between lower socio-economic status and perinatal mortality, intrauterine growth retardation, congenital malformations and mental retardation were shown by WILKERSON et al. (1966), DRILLIEN (1967), BANERJEE (1969) and NAEYE et al. (1969). Generally, undernourishment during pregnancy is thought to be the responsible factor. Mental retardation also is often thought to be due to socio-cultural deficiencies. In our opinion the possible role of ovopathy is under-estimated in this respect since accompanying congenital deviations (DRILLIEN 1967) cannot be explained by socio-cultural factors alone. An increase in twin pregnancies in mothers from lower socio-economic classes (LIN and CHEN 1968) too, points towards factors influencing the ovulatory process.

10. Failures during application of the calendar rhythmic method (including weekend marriages)

In two retrospective investigations a significant increase of abnormal progeny was found in couples applying the calendar rhythmic method (JONGBLOET 1969 and 1970). On purely theoretical grounds weekend marriages might enhance the chances of abnormal progeny, as the possibility of intratubal overripeness might thereby be increased.

11. Conceptions under emotional stress
The possibility of psychological influences on the menstrual cycle and ovulation is well established. Therefore it is to be expected that under stress situations, where ovulation is temporarily inhibited, overripeness ovopathy will increase.

12. Conceptions during treatment with drugs which can postpone ovulation (psychopharmaca, antihypertensiva and barbiturates)
We formerly suggested (JONGBLOET 1969 and 1970) that, in analogy with animal experiments, drugs which reduce the monoamino reserves in the hypothalamus, can hamper or even interrupt the process of ovulation. Such inhibition might conceivably increase the chances of intrafollicular overripeness of the egg.

CRITERION VIII: MALFORMATIONS CAUSED BY OVERRIPENESS OVOPATHY ARE RELATIVELY MORE FREQUENTLY ACCOMPANIED BY COMPLICATIONS OF PREGNANCY, BIRTH AND NEONATAL LIFE

Through the whole literature concerning causes of mental and physical handicaps, the high frequency of complications during pregnancy, parturition and neonatal life, are continually recurring themes. The more these complications concern late pregnancy, birth or the neonatal period, the more it is evident that the child was in distress. That is probably the reason why the belief that these complications are the primary cause of later handicaps is widespread, although several critical researchworkers have thrown their doubts on this common assumption. The question has been raised how indeed these late pregnancy complications, obstetric factors and perinatal distress could explain cerebral malformations, congenital anomalies and abnormal dermatoglyphs, structures which must develop at a very early stage of pregnancy (JONGBLOET 1970). IFFY (1961, 1962, 1963 and 1968) thought that post-mid-cycle-conceptions might cause a higher incidence of tubal pregnancies, mola hydatidosa and abortions. Overripeness ovopathy, therefore, as a primary cause of developmental malformations and particularly of chromosomal aberrations, might enhance associated complications of pregnancy, parturition and neonatal life. The following arguments favour this line of thought:

a Many of these complications occur more frequently in the above mentioned 'high risk' conception groups such as adolescent girls, primiparous and premenopausal women (STILL 1927, CANZLER et al. 1969, NITZSCHE and

WIENOLD 1969, COATES 1970 and FRANCIS 1970), (pre)diabetic women (NAVARRETE 1970), after a very short or a long unintended conception interval (AREY 1923, CHABERT et al. 1970), and especially during spring and autumn (EUFINGER and WEIKERSHEIMER 1933, PASAMANICK and KNOBLOCH 1958, TIMONEN et al. 1965).

b Many of these complications occur more frequently together with chromosomal aberrations. The association between pregnancy complications such as vaginal blood loss or placenta praevia and congenital, let alone chromosomal, aberrations, is difficult to explain as a causal relationship. It is more probable that both are the result of a common cause such as a functionally suboptimal, c.q. overripe, egg.

c Many of these complications occur more frequently in multiple pregnancies. Fertilization of two different eggs, instead of one, might indicate a disturbance in the pattern of follicle ripening. Multiple pregnancies indeed are more frequently seen in elderly mothers (GEDDA and BRENCI 1968), after conceptions in spring and autumn (TIMONEN and CARPEN 1968), after a long pregnancy interval (WYSHAK 1969), after stopping oral contraceptives (WATTS et al. 1964) and also in socio-economic lower classes (LIN and CHEN 1968). Such increase suggests a more or less synchronous ripening and bursting of several follicles, due to an imbalanced hormonal regulation. Thus, ovulations occurring at different moments could lead to superfecundation and even superfoetation, respectively to fertilization of two egg cells during the same cycle or during consecutive cycles.

d Finally, several of these complications tend to occur in combination. The developing embryo indeed forms a functional unit with placenta, membranes and umbilical cord. Damage of the egg in this respect might thus lead to abnormal adnexae, abnormal implantation and other complications.

Some of the complications concerned are particularly interesting, *viz.*

– *ectopic pregnancy and placenta praevia*
IFFY's reflux theory assumes that an ovum liberated just before menstruation cannot be sufficiently implanted in time and can be displaced by the mechanical effect of the menstrual flow. The latter could drive the insufficiently implanted blastocyst back into one of the tubes or even into the abdomen. On the other hand, it could also take it along to the cervix uteri. By this mechanism tubal and abdominal pregnancy could be explained on the one hand and placenta praevia, placenta marginalis and cervical implantation on the other. MALL (1908) found that in extra-uterine pregnancies 65% of the embryos showed malformations. About half of these concerned the C.N.S. Next, congenital malformations are often associated with placenta praevia, as mentioned by GREENHILL (1939), RECORD and MCKEOWN (1949), SMILKSTEIN (1962) and others

who found a marked increase of placenta praevia in anencephaly. In the case of trisomy 21 there are also indications that an aberrant implantation occurs more often than normal (BENDA 1969).

The combination of a handicapped child and ante partum haemorrhage or dystocia caused by placenta marginalis and placenta praevia might easily lead to false conclusions. For, if the child happens to be born with mental or neurological handicaps there is a tendency to ascribe these rather to the difficulties during delivery than to the underlying common cause mentioned above.

– vaginal blood loss during pregnancy, and threatening abortion
If the first menstruation after conception is not entirely suppressed, as might be the case in late liberation of the egg cell, false interpretation of the length of pregnancy can be expected. BATTAGLIA et al. (1966) drew attention to this group of children with so called 'high birth weight-low gestational age' who are too heavy in relation to the ostensible length of pregnancy. They found this to be a 'high risk' group with a perinatal mortality five times higher than normal. WIENER (1970) moreover noticed retarded mental development in this group of children. In the framework of the overripeness theory the poor prognosis of these children should not be ascribed to the vaginal bleeding itself, but to fertilization of an overripe egg. These children, in other words should not be judged too heavy for their real intrauterine age, and the term 'high birth weight-low gestational age' should be abandoned.

Both prospective and retrospective investigations have established that vaginal bleeding occurs more frequently during pregnancies ending in abortion, still-birth or birth of a child with malformations (LANDTMAN 1948, TURNBULL and WALKER 1956, McDONALD 1958 and 1961, SHAPIRO et al. 1965 and WILKERSON et al. 1966).

– abortion, intra-uterine death, still-birth and premature birth
NISHIMURA (1966 and 1969) found that congenital and chromosomal aberrations in embryos delivered by therapeutic abortion were far more frequent (10 to 100 times) than in newly born children. He therefore concluded that many of these embryos with anencephaly, myeloschizis, palatocheiloschizis, polydactyly, hermaphroditism and various chromosomal aberrations would have aborted spontaneously later on. Studies concerning spontaneous abortion, indeed, confirm these suspicions. A marked increase in developmental anomalies in abortus products was stated by POLAND (1968) and MIKAMO (1970), while CARR (1967) and BOUÉ and BOUÉ (1969) found trisomy G in respectively 3 % and 10 % of spontaneous abortions. Also, in late foetal and neonatal deaths, more malformations are found than in surviving children. MASTER-NOTANI et al. (1968) in a prospective investigation, observed developmental defects in 1.02% of live-borns and in 9.45%, resp. 9.24% of still-births, resp. perinatal

deaths. HEDBERG et al. (1963) found the perinatal mortality among malformed children to be 9.6% as against 1.6% in a control group. Among premature children (or rather children with a birth weight of 2.500 grammes or under) they found 11% malformations, as against 4% in a control group.

– intrauterine growth retardation
DRILLIEN (1968) studied thoroughly the causes of handicap in low birth weight infants and concluded that the primary cause of later disability is developmental malformation and that low birth weight and/or premature labour are secondary to this. Therefore low birth weight, c.q. prematurity, might not be the primary cause of later handicap. This primary cause of intra-uterine growth retardation has, in our opinion, to be sought rather in overripeness ovopathy, since the phenomenon answers most of the above mentioned criteria.

– hydramnios and toxaemia
Hydramnios often occurs in combination with toxaemia, and is regularly accompanied by abnormalities of placenta and foetus. PRINDLE et al. (1955) considered these association as 'manifestations of the same maternal disease'.

REVIEW

The criteria for possible overripeness ovopathy discussed in the foregoing have been derived from and tested against data from the literature and personal data. The results are shown in tables 2, 3, 4 and 5 for Down's syndrome, congenital aberrations of the C.N.S., palatocheiloschizis and congenital hip disease. Generally speaking, they tend to suggest that these malformations can be the result of overripeness ovopathy. Juvenile myxoedema or cretinism and DiGeorge's syndrome also answer many of the above mentioned criteria, but because of their rare occurrence convincing data are still lacking.

These criteria could be applied to other chromosomal aberrations, to malformations of the cardiovascular, urogenital, intestinal and skeletal systems, and to various forms of cancerous processes, psychopathology and morphological deviations of eyes, ears, face and extremities, in order to find out whether, and if so, to what extent, these diseases, too, might be the result of overripeness ovopathy.

However, it remains important to separate on the one hand the genocopies caused by genetic factors and on the other hand the phenocopies caused by peristatic factors. Thus, Down's syndrome with translocation is, strictly speaking a genocopy of the classical trisomy G. Using the first criterion the two can be usually separated, since Down's syndrome with translocation occurs familially, while classical trisomy G does not or only very rarely. Conse-

TABLE 5

	VIII RELATIVELY MORE FREQUENTLY ACCOMPANIED BY COMPLICATIONS OF PREGNANCY,				
	Ectopic pregnancy and placenta praevia	Vaginal blood loss and threatening abortion	Abortion and intrauterine death	Still-birth	Praemature birth (duration of pregnancy)
Down's syndrome	Benda 1949 Benda 1969	Geyer 1941 Ingalls 1947 Benda 1949 Oster 1953 Ingalls et al. 1957 Cowie et al. 1968	Carr 1967 Boué et al. 1969 Nishimura 1969	Buchan 1962 Record et al. 1955 Chen et al. 1970	Buchan 1962 Marmol et al. 1969
Anencephaly, meningo-myelocoele, spina bifida	Mall 1908 Greenhill 1939 Record et al. 1949 Smilkstein 1962	Record et al.1949 Smithells et al. 1965	Poland 1968 Nishimura 1969 Milic 1969	Frézal et al. 1964 all reviews concerning this subject	Frézal et al. 1964 Milic 1969 Milic et al. 1969
Palatoschizis and palatocheiloschizis		Drillien et al. 1966 Fraser 1970	Nishimura 1969	Drillien et al. 1966	Bethman 1969 Bardanouve 1969
Congenital hip disease	Record et al. 1958	Illyés 1969			
Agenesis and dysgenesis of thyroid gland					
Dysgenesis of thymus and/or parathyroid glands (DiGeorge syndrome)					

				of PARTURITION	and of NEONATAL LIFE
Intrauterine growth retardation	Toxaemia	Hydramnios	Delayed parturition and dysmaturity		
Smith et al. 1955 Ingalls et al. 1957 Tonomura et al. 1966 Marmol et al. 1969 Chen et al. 1969	Beidleman 1945 Cowie et al. 1968 Canzler et al. 1969	Prindle et al. 1955 Cowie et al. 1968			Oster 1953 Record et al. 1955
Milic 1969 Cassady 1969 Milic ot al. 1969	Erez 1966 Canzler et al. 1969	Smilkstein 1962 Prindle et al. 1955 Comerford 1965 Smithells et al. 1965 Erez et al. 1966	Frézal 1964 Milic et al. 1969	Comerford 1965 Erez et al. 1966	Record et al. 1949
Drillien et al. 1966 Bethman 1969 Bardanouve 1969	Fraser 1970 Canzler et al. 1970		Drillien et al. 1966	Drillien et al. 1966 Gilmore et al. 1966	Drillien et al. 1966 Bardanouve 1969
Record et al. 1958	Record et al. 1958			Record et al. 1958 Nagura 1960 Woolf et al. 1968	

quently, both forms of Down's syndrome should differ in all other criteria also. So, for instance, it is known that the occurrence of Down's syndrome with translocation is not correlated with the age of the mother.

A second example is palatocheiloschizis. DRILLIEN et al. (1966) encountered many of the above criteria in a 'non-familial cleft lip and palate' group, while they were absent in the familial, *i.e.* presumably the inheritable groups. Therefore, the latter are genocopies. A similar malformation, however occurring after rubella or thalidomide during pregnancy (FRASER 1970) should then be considered a phenocopy. A third example of the distinction between the results of ovopathy and genocopies are the dysgeneses of thyroid and of thymus and parathyroid glands; the former occur sporadically, in contrast to the latter which are inherited autosomally or sex-linked. Used in this way the 'overripeness criteria' cited might be of great help in nosological classification.

SUMMARY

After it was shown that overripeness ovopathy is important as a teratologic factor in man (JONGBLOET 1968, 1969, 1970, 1971a, b and c) criteria were formulated, which a malformation or a chromosomal aberration has to satisfy to make overripeness ovopathy acceptable as aetiology.

Malformations and other diseases, caused by overripeness ovopathy, have to satisfy the following criteria:

I.   They do not or only very rarely occur familially;
II. They frequently occur in both monozygotic twins of equal size, but more especially only in the smaller one of such a twin pair;
III. They are often accompanied by a multiplicity of congenital malformations, including 'idiopathic' mental retardation and 'degenerative' stigmata;
IV. They are often accompanied by non-specific chromosomal aberrations;
V.   They are often characterized by hypogonadism;
VI. They are often a symptom of a maternal constitutional factor, which manifests itself in a suboptimal reproductive history;
VII. They occur relatively frequently with 'high risk' conceptions;
VIII. They are relatively more frequently accompanied by complications of pregnancy, parturition and neonatal life.

Using these criteria various malformations were studied, such as Down's syndrome, congenital malformations of the C.N.S., palatocheiloschizis, congenital hip disease, dysgenesis of thyroid, thymus and parathyroid glands (DiGeorge's syndrome). For all these anomalies arguments were found making overripeness ovopathy acceptable as an aetiological factor. By means of these 'overripeness criteria' genocopies (caused by hereditary factors) and pheno-copies (caused by peristatic factors) can sometimes be distinguished from aberrations caused by overripeness ovopathy. This offers a better outlook in counselling parents, in prophylaxis and eventually in treatment of the mother.

SAMENVATTING

Nadat werd aangetoond dat de overrijpingsovopathie als teratologische faktor ook bij de mens van belang is (JONGBLOET 1968, 1969, 1970, 1971a, b en c) werden criteria geformuleerd, waaraan een ontwikkelingsstoornis of een chromosomale afwijking moet voldoen om overrijpingsovopathie als etiologie aannemelijk te maken.

Misvormingen en andere ziektebeelden, door overrijpingsovopathie ver-oorzaakt, moeten voldoen aan de volgende criteria:

I. Zij komen niet dan hoogst zelden familiaal voor;
II. Zij komen frekwent voor bij monozygote tweelingen van gelijke grootte, maar vooral bij de kleinere helft van een dergelijk tweelingpaar;
III. Zij worden meestal begeleid door veelsoortige congenitale afwijkingen, waaronder 'idiopathische' mentale retardatie en 'degeneratieve af-wijkingen';
IV. Zij gaan vaak gepaard met niet-specifieke chromosomale afwijkingen;
V. Zij gaan veelal gepaard met hypogonadisme;
VI. Zij zijn dikwijls symptoom van een moederlijke constitutionele faktor die zich o.m. kan uiten in een verminderde voortplantingsmogelijkheid;
VII. Zij plegen frekwenter voor te komen na 'high risk' concepties;
VIII. Zij gaan dikwijls gepaard met komplikaties in de zwangerschap, tijdens de bevalling en in de neonatale periode.

Verscheidene afwijkingen werden aan de hand van deze criteria onderzocht, zoals het syndroom van Down, congenitale misvormingen van het C.Z.S., pala-tocheiloschizis, congenitale heupdysplasie en -luxatie, dysgenesis van schild-klier, thymus en bijschildklieren (syndroom van DiGeorge). Voor al deze afwijkingen bleek een grote congruentie te bestaan van argumenten die pleiten voor overrijpingsovopathie als etiologie. Aan de hand van deze overrijpings-criteria zouden genocopieën (endogeen) en fenocopieën (door peristatische faktoren) kunnen worden onderscheiden van 'overrijpingsovopathieën'. Hier-door zou de 'counselling' der ouders, de prophylaxis en de eventuele behande-ling van de moeder kunnen worden verbeterd.

ACKNOWLEDGMENT

We would especially like to thank Prof. Dr. T. D. Stahlie, paediatrician, Free University of Amsterdam and Dr. J. V. T. H. Hamerlynck, Department of Obstetrics and Gynaecology, Wilhelmina Gasthuis, University of Amsterdam, for their critical remarks and fruitful discussions. The tables were composed by Miss A. M. A. Verstraaten and the translation was carried out by Dr. J. A. M. and Mrs. G. A. van der Mey, B.Sc. We thank them for their coöperation.

REFERENCES

AREY, L. B., Tubal twins and tubal pregnancy. *Surg. Gynec. Obstet.* 36: 803, 1923.

BANERJEE, P., Birth weight of the Bengali newborn: effect of the economic position of the mother. *Ann. hum. Genet.* 33: 99, 1969.

BARDANOUVE, V. T., Cleft palate in Montana. A 10 year report. *Cleft Palate J.*, 6: 213, 1969.

BATTAGLIA, F. C., T. M. FRAZIER and A. E. HELLEGERS, Birth weight, gestational age and pregnancy outcome with special reference to high birth weight-low gestational age infant. *Pediatrics* 37: 417, 1966.

BEARN, J. G., Anencephaly and the development of the male genital tract. *Acta Paediat. Acad. Sc. Hung.* 9: 159, 1968.

BEIDLEMAN, B., Mongolism: a selective review. *Amer. J. ment. Defic.* 50: 35, 1945.

BELLEFEUILLE, P. DE, Contribution à l'étiologie de l'anencéphalie par l'étude des jumeaux. *Un. méd. Can.* 98: 438, 1969.

BENDA, C. E., Prenatal maternal factors in mongolism. *J. Amer. med. Ass.* 139: 979, 1949.

BENDA, C. E., *Down's Syndrome.* Mongolism and its management. Grune & Stratton, New York-London, 1969.

BETHMAN, W. and J. EIFERT, Die Häufigkeit der Frühgeborenen unter den Tragern von Lippen-Kiefer-Gaumensegel Spalten. *Dtsch. Stomat.* 19: 649, 1969.

BORÇBAKAN, C., An analysis of 1.000 cases of cleft lip and palate in Turkey. *Cleft Palate J.* 6: 210,1969.

BOUÉ, J. G. and A. BOUÉ, Fréquence des aberrations chromosomiques dans les avortements spontanés humains. *C. R. Acad. Sci. (Paris)* 269: 283, 1969.

BRUNNER, E. K., The outcome of 1556 conceptions. A medical and sociological study. *Hum. Biol.* 13: 159, 1941.

BUCHAN, L. R., A study of mongolism in Newcastle-upon-Tyne 1948—1959. *Med. Offr.* 107: 51, 1962.

BUCK, C., G. H. VALENTINE and K. HAMILTON, A study of microsymptoms in the parents and sibs of patients with Down's syndrome. *Amer. J. ment. Defic.* 73: 683, 1969.

CAMPBELL, M., Causes of malformations of heart. *Brit. med. J.* 2: 895, 1965.

CANZLER, E., G. FUNK and L. SCHLEGEL, Die Missbildungshäufigkeit an der Universitäts-Frauenklinik Leipzig in den Jahren 1941 bis 1965. I and II. *Zbl. Gynak* 26: 833 and 847.

CARR, D. H., Chromosome anomalies as a cause of spontaneous abortion. *Amer. J. Obstet. Gynec.* 97: 283, 1967.

CARTER, C. O., K. M. LAURENCE and P. A. DAVID, Genetics of major central nervous system malformations, based on South Wales socio-genetic investigation. *Dev. Med. Child. Neurol.* 9: Suppl. 13, 30, 1967.

CARTER, C. O., Spina bifida and anencephaly: A problem in genetic-environmental interaction. *J. Biosoc. Sci.* 1: 71, 1969.

CASSADY, G., Anencephaly: A 6-year study of 367 cases. *Amer. J. Obstet. Gynec.* 103: 1154, 1969.

CECCARELLI, G. and L. TORBIDONI, Le malformazioni associate alla sindrome di Down. *Pediatria* 5: 708, 1968.

CHABERT, P., J. SUAUDEAU, CL.RACINET et al., A propos d'une série de 141 grossesse extra-utérines. *Rev. franç. Gynéc.* 65: 249, 1970.

CHEN, A. T. L., F. R. SERGOVICH, J. S. McKIM et al., Chromosome studies in full-term, low-birth-weight, mentally retarded patients. *J. Pediat.* 76: 393, 1970.

CHIERI, R. A., O. H. PIVETTA and V. G. FOGLIA, Altered ovulation pattern in experimental diabetes. *Fertil. and Steril.* 20: 661, 1969.

CHRISTAKOS, A. C. and J. L. SIMPSON, Anencephaly in three siblings. *Obstet. and Gynec.* 33: 267, 1969.

COATES, J. B., Obstetrics in the very young adolescent. *Amer. J. Obstet. Gynec.* 108: 68, 1970.

CODACCIONI, J. L., H. RUF and P. BROCHERY, Pré-diabète et grossesse. *Marseille méd.* 106: 797, 1969.

COFFEY, V. P. and W. J. E. JESSOP, A study of 137 cases of anencephaly. *Brit. J. prev. soc. Med.* 11: 174, 1957.

COMERFORD, J. B., Pregnancy with anencephaly. *Lancet i:* 679, 1965.

COWIE, V. and E. SLATER, The fertility of mothers of mongols. *J. ment. Defic. Res.* 12: 196, 1968.

CROSS, R. G., Anencephalus and spina bifida. *Brit. Med. J.* 3: 253, 1968.

DALLAIRE, L., D. KINGSMILL-FLYNN and G. LEBOEUF, Autoimmunity and chromosomal aberrations. *Canad. med. Ass. J.* 100: 1, 1969.

DODSON, W. E., D. ALEXANDER, M. AL-AISH et al., The DiGeorge syndrome. *Lancet i:* 574, 1969.

DOWN, L., Discussion. *Brit. Med. J.* 2: 665, 1909.

DRILLIEN, C. M., T. T. S. INGRAM and E. M. WILKINSON, *The causes and natural history of cleft lip and palate.* Livingstone, Edinburgh, 1966.

DRILLIEN, C. M., *Proceed. of the first congress of the international Association for the Scientific study of mental deficiency* (Montpellier). B. W. Richards, Michael Jackson Publ. C. L., 1967, p. 113.

DRILLIEN, C. M., *Aspects of praematurity and dysmaturity.* Nutricia Symposium (Groningen). H. E. Stenfert Kroese N.V., 1968, p. 287.

EREZ, S. and T. M. KING, Anencephaly: a survey of 44 cases. *Obstet. and Gynec.* 27: 601, 1966.

EUFINGER, H. and J. WEIKERSHEIMER, Der Einfluss atmosphärischer Vorgänge auf Eklampsieausbruch. *Arch. Gynäk.* 154: 15, 1933.

FABIA, J. and M. DROLETTE, Malformations and leukemia in children with Down's syndrome. *Pediatrics* 45: 60, 1970.

FEDRICK, J., Anencephalus: variation with maternal age, parity, social class and region in England, Scotland and Wales. *Ann. hum. Genet. (Lond.)* 34: 31, 1970.

FERM, V. H., Conjoined twinning in mammalian teratology. *Arch. environm. Hlth.* 19: 353, 1969.

FIALKOW, P. J., Autoimmunity: a predisposing factor to chromosomal aberrations? *Lancet i:* 474, 1964.

FIALKOW, P. J., Autoantibodies and chromosomal aberrations. *Lancet i:* 1106, 1967.

FRANCIS, W. J. A., Reproduction at menarche and menopause in women. *J. Reprod. Fertill.,* Suppl. 12: 89, 1970.

FRASER, F. C., The genetics of cleft lip and cleft palate. *Amer. J. hum. Genet.* 22: 336, 1970.

FREZAL, J., J. KELLEY, M. L. GUILLEMOT et al., Anencephaly in France. *Amer. J. hum. Genet.* 16: 336, 1964.

GEDDA, L. and G. BRENCI, Fertility and multiple births. *A. Ge. Me. Ge.* 17: 417, 1968.

GERMAN, J., Mongolism, delayed fertilization and human sexual behavior. *Nature* 217: 516, 1968.

GEYER, H., Die Insuffizienz der Ovarien bei Müttern von Mongoloiden. *Z. ges. Neurol. Psychiat.* 173: 47, 1941.

GILMORE, S. I. and S. M. HOFMAN, Clefts in Wisconsin, incidence and related factors. *Cleft Palate J.* 3: 186, 1966.

GITHENS, J. H., F. MUSCHENHEIM, V. A. FULGINITI et al., Thymic alymphoplasia with XX/XY lymphoid chimerism secondary to probable maternal-fetal transfusion. *J. Pediat.* 75: 87, 1969.

GORDON, H., D. DAVIES, V. BOTHA et al., Cleft lip-palate in Cape Town. *S. Afr. med. J.* 43: 1267, 1969.

GREENBERG, R. C., Two factors influencing the births of mongols to younger mothers. *Med. Offr.* 109: 62, 1963.

GREENHILL, J. P., The increased incidence of fetal abnormalities in cases of placenta previa. *Amer. J. Obstet. Gynec.* 37: 624, 1939.

141

GREIG, W. R., A. S. HENDERSON, J. A. BOYLE et al., Thyroid dysgenesis in two pairs of monozygotic twins and in a mother and child. *J. Clin. Endocr.* 26: 1309, 1966.

GROOT, M. J. W. DE, Epidemiologische aspecten van de aangeboren misvormingen. *Huisarts en wetenschap* 8: 121, 1965. Ibidem 176. Ibidem 211.

HALBERTSMA, T., Over mongoloïde idiotie, naar aanleiding van een aantal gevallen bij tweelingen. *Ned. T. Geneesk.* 66: 22, 1922.

HAMERSMA, K., *Anencephalie en spina bifida.* Drukkerij Romijn, Apeldoorn, 1966.

HECHT, F., J. S. BRYANT, A. G. MOTULSKY et al., The no. 17-18 (E) trisomy syndrome: Studies on cytogenetics, dermatoglyphics, paternal age and linkage. *J. Pediat.* 63: 605, 1963.

HECHT, F., J. E. NIEVAARD, N. DUNCANSON et al., Double aneuploidy: the frequency of XYY in males with Down's syndrome. *Amer. J. hum. Genet.* 21: 352, 1969.

HEDBERG, E., K. HOLMDAHL, S. PEHRSON et al., On relationship between maternal conditions during pregnancy and congenital malformations. *Acta paediat.* 52: 353, 1963.

HENDRICKS, CH. H., Congenital malformations. *Obstet. and Gynec.* 6: 592, 1955.

HOLLAND, W. W., R. DOLL and C. O. CARTER, The mortality from leukaemia and other cancers among patients with Down's syndrome and among their parents. *Brit. J. Cancer* 16: 177, 1962.

HOROWITZ, J. and A. McDONALD, Anencephaly and spina bifida in the Province of Quebec. *Canad. Med. Ass. J.* 100: 748, 1969.

IFFY, L., Contribution to the aetiology of ectopic pregnancy. *J. Obstet. Gynaec. Brit. Cwlth.* 68: 441, 1961.

IFFY, L., Contribution to the aetiology of hydatidiform mole. *Ann. Chir. Gyn. Fenn.* 51: 428, 1962.

IFFY, L. and P. KERNER, The aetiology of early abortion. *J. Obstet. Gynaec. Brit. Cwlth.* 69: 598, 1962.

IFFY, L., The role of premenstrual, post-midcycle conception in the aetiology of ectopic gestation. *J. Obstet. Gynaec. Brit. Cwlth.* 70: 996, 1963.

IFFY, L., The time of conception in pathological gestations. *Proc. Roy. Soc. Med.* 56: 1098, 1963.

IFFY, L., Recent investigations concerning the aetiology of ectopic pregnancies. *Aust. N. Z. J. Obstet. Gynaec.* 8: 131, 1968.

ILLYÉS, Zs., Die Rolle der exogenen Schäden bei der Entstehung der angeborenen Hüftluxation und -dysplasie. *Beitr. Orthop. Traum.* 15: 453, 1968.

ILLYÉS, Zs., Zusammenhang von Vererbung und exogenen Schädigungen bei der Entstehung von Luxation und Dysplasia coxae congenita. *Beitr. Orthop. Traum.* 16: 3, 1969.

INGALLS, TH. H., Etiology of mongolism. *Amer. J. Dis. Child.* 74: 147, 1947.

INGALLS, TH. H., J. BABBOTT and R. PHILBROOK, The mothers of mongoloid babies: A retrospective appraisal of their health during pregnancy. *Amer. J. Obstet. Gynec.* 74: 572, 1957.

INGALLS, TH. H., R. PHILBROOK and A. MAJIMA, Conjoined twins in zebra fish. *Arch. Environm. Hlth* 19: 344, 1969.

JAMES, W. H., Still birth, neonatal death and birth interval. *Ann. hum. Genet.* London 32: 163, 1968.

JONGBLOET, P. H., Overripeness of the egg. *Maandschr. Kindergeneesk.* 36: 352, 1968.

JONGBLOET, P. H., The intriguing phenomenon of gametopathy and its disastrous effects on the human progeny. *Maandschr. Kindergeneesk.* 37: 261, 1969.

JONGBLOET, P. H., An investigation into the occurrence of overripeness ovopathy in the normal population. With coöperation of A. Arends, Y. Margry and M. Strankinga. *Maandschr. Kindergeneesk.* 38: 228, 1970.

JONGBLOET, P. H. and G. M. PACILLY, De samenhang tussen maand van geboorte en gametopathie. *Ned. T. Psychiat.* 13: 98, 1971.

JONGBLOET, P. H., Month of birth and gametopathy. *Clin. Genet.* 2: 1971 (a).

JONGBLOET, P. H., Status Bonnevie-Ullrich and Turner's syndrome. Overripeness ovopathy as a unifying concept. Part I and II. In: *Mental and physical handicaps in connection with overripeness ovopathy.* H. E. Stenfert Kroese N.V., Leiden, 1971 (b and c).

KADOWAKI, J., R. I. THOMPSON, W. W. ZUELZER et al., XX/XY lymphoid chimaerism in congenital immunological deficiency syndrome with thymic alymphoplasia. *Lancet* ii: 1152, 1965.

KARASOVÁ, M., A case of monozygote twins with triple discordancy in the system of papillary V R and U factors. *Bratisl. Lek. Listy* 51: 86, 1969.

KAUFMANN, H. J. and W. F. TAILLARD, Pelvic abnormalities in mongols. *Brit. Med. J.* 1: 948, 1961.

KLEBANOW, D., Hunger und psychische Erregungen als Ovar- und Keimschädigungen. *Geburtsh. u. Frauenheilk.* 7/8: 812, 1948.

KLEIN, H. J. and R. FISCHER, Embryopathia diabetica. *Med. Welt* 47: 2621, 1968.

KRETSCHMER, R., B. SAY, D. BROWN et al., Congenital aplasia of the thymus gland (DiGeorge's syndrome). *New Engl. J. Med.* 279: 1295, 1968.

LANDE-CHAMPAIN, L., The etiology of mongolism. *J. Child Psychiat.* 3: 53, 1954.

LANDTMAN, B., On the relationship between maternal conditions during pregnancy and congenital malformations. *Arch. Dis. Childh.* 23: 237, 1948.

LAURENCE, K. M., C. O. CARTER and P. A. DAVID, Major central nervous system malformations in South Wales. *Brit. J. prev. soc. Med.* 22: 212, 1968.

LEJEUNE, J., Etudes des chromosomes-somatiques de neuf enfants mongoliens. *C. R. Acad. Sci.* 248: 1721, 1959.

LEPRAT, J. and J. C. VALCKE, L'hypothyroïdie de l'adulte. *Presse Méd.* 77: 119, 1969.

LIN, R. S. and K. P. CHEN, A preliminary twin study in Taiwan. I. Epidemiological aspect. *J. Formosan Med. Ass.* 67: 329, 1968.

LISCHNER, H. W. and A. M. DIGEORGE, Role of thymus in humoral immunity. *Lancet* ii: 1044, 1969.

LORMANS-LAUWERS, S., C. VAN KEMPEN, A. HAMERS et al., Hypofysaire hypothyreoidie bij een patiente met trisomie X. *Maandschr. Kindergeneesk.* 38: 161, 1970.

LUNN, J. E., A survey of mongol children in Glasgow. *Scot. med. J.* 4: 368, 1959.

McDONALD, A. D., Maternal health and congenital defect; a prospective investigation. *New Engl. J. Med.* 258: 767, 1958.

McDONALD, A. D., Maternal health in early pregnancy and congenital defect. *Brit. J. prev. soc. Med.* 15: 154, 1961.

McGIRR, E. M. and J. H. HUTCHISON, Dysgenesis of the thyroid gland as a cause of cretinism and juvenile myxedema. *J. Clin. Endocr.* 15: 668, 1955.

MACMAHON, B. and S. YEN, Unrecognised epidemic of anencephaly and spina bifida. *Lancet* i: 31, 1971.

McNEIL, TH. F., R. WIEGERINK and J. E. DOZIER, Pregnancy and birth complications in the births of seriously, moderately and mildly behaviorally disturbed children. *J. Nerv. Ment. Dis.* 151: 24, 1970.

MALKANI, P. K. and J. J. MIRCHANDANI, Menstruation during lactation. *J. Obstet. Gynec. (India)* 11: 11, 1960.

MALL, F. P., Origin of human monsters. *J. Morph.* 19: 3, 1908.

MARKOVIC, M. D., Conjoined twins with mirror-image clefts of lip and palate. *Cleft Palate J.* 7: 690, 1970.

MARMOL, J. G., A. L. SCRIGGINS and R. F. VOLLMAN, Mothers of mongoloid infants in the collaborative project. *Amer. J. Obstet. Gynec.* 104: 533, 1969.

MASTER-NOTANI, P., P. J. KOLAH and L. D. SANGHVI, Congenital malformations in the newborn in Bombay. *Acta genet. (Basel)* 18: 193, 1968.

MATSUNAGA, E., Parental age, live-birth order and pregnancy-free interval in Down's syndrome in Japan. In: *Mongolism*, Ciba Foundation Study Group No. 25, Little, Brown and Company, Boston 1967, p. 6.

MENSER, M. A. and S. G. PURVIS-SMITH, Dermatoglyphic defects in children with leukaemia. *Lancet* i: 1076, 1969.

MESKIN, L. H. and S. PRUZANSKY, A malformation profile of facial cleft patients and their siblings. *Cleft Palate J.* 6: 309, 1969.

MIKAMO, K., Intrafollicular overripeness and teratologic development. *Cytogenetics* 7: 212, 1968.

MIKAMO, K., Anatomic and chromosomal anomalies in spontaneous abortion. *Amer. J. Obstet. Gynec.* 106: 243, 1970.

MILIC, A. B. and K. ADAMSONS, The relationship between anencephaly and prolonged pregnancy. *J. Obstet. Gynaec. Brit. Cwlth.* 76: 102, 1969.

MILIC, A. B., The occurrence of anencephaly at the Sloane Hospital for Women 1942–1967. *Bulletin of the Sloane Hospital for women* 15: 11, 1969.

MILUNSKY, A., Glucose intolerance in the parents of children with Down's syndrome. *Amer. J. Ment. Defic.* 74: 475, 1970.

MORISON, J. E., Congenital malformations in one of monozygotic twins. *Arch. Dis. Childh.* 24: 214, 1949.

MYRIANTHOPOULOS, N. C., Role of maternal factors in the occurrence of congenital malformations and other abnormalities of childhood. 3rd International conference on congenital malformations. The Hague. *Excerpta medica International Congress Series* nr. 191: 66, 1969.

NAEYE, R. L., Organ abnormalities in a human parabiotic syndrome. *Amer. J. Pathol.* 46: 829, 1965.

NAEYE, R. L., M. M. DIENER, W. J. DELLINGER et al., Urban poverty: Effects on prenatal nutrition. *Science* 166: 1026, 1969.

NAGURA, S., Zur Frage der Vererbung der angeborenen Hüftverrenkung. *Zbl. Chir.* 85: 2167, 1960.

NANCE, W. E., Anencephaly and spina bifida: a possible example of cytoplasmic inheritance in man. *Nature* 224: 373, 1969.

NAVARRETE, V. N., H. E. PANIAGUA, C. R. ALGER et al. ,The significance of metabolic adjustment before a new pregnancy. *Amer. J. Obst. Gynec.* 107: 250, 1970.

NAVARRETE, V. N., C. E. ROJAS, C. R. ALGER et al., Subsequent diabetes in mothers delivered of a malformed infant. *Lancet* ii: 993, 1970.

NEWMAN, H. H., Organic symmetry in armadillo quadruplets. *Biol. Bull.* 30: 173, 1916.

NIELSEN, J., Inheritance in monozygotic twins. *Lancet* ii: 717, 1967.

NISHIMURA, H., K. TAKANO, T. TANIMURA et al., High incidence of several malformations in the early human embryos as compared with infants. *Biol. Neonat.* 10: 93, 1966.

NISHIMURA, H., Incidence of malformations in abortions. Congenital malformations. Proceedings of the 3rd International Conference, The Hague, *Excerpta Med.*, Amsterdam-New York, 1969.

NITZSCHE, P. and J. WIENOLD, Schwangerschaft, Geburt und Wochenbett bei Jugendlichen. *Zbl. Gynäk.* 91: 348, 1969.

NYLANDER, P. P. S., The determination of zygosity. A study of 608 pairs of twins born in Aberdeen. *J. Obstet. Gynaec. Brit. Cwlth.* 77: 506, 1970.

ØSTER, J., *Mongolism*. Danish Sc. Press Ltd., Copenhagen, 1953.

PANNBACKER, M., Congenital malformations and cleft lip and palate. *Cleft Palate J.* 5: 334, 1968.

PASAMANICK, B. and H. KNOBLOCH, Seasonal variation in complications of pregnancy. *J. Obstet. Gynaec.* 12: 110, 1958.

PENROSE, L. S., The distal triradius t on the hands of parents and sibs of mongol imbeciles. *Ann. hum. Genet.* 19: 10, 1954.

PENROSE, L. S., Genetics of anencephaly. *J. ment. Defic. Res.* 1: 4, 1957.

PENROSE, L. S. and G. F. SMITH, *Down's anomaly*. J. & A. Churchill Ltd., London, 1966.

PERGAMENT, E., G. C. PIETRA, T. KADOTANI et al., A ring chromosome no. 16 in an infant with primary hypoparathyroidism. *J. Pediat.* 76: 745, 1970.

PETERS, A. and W. CULLEY, Urinary levels of testosterone and epitestosterone in Down's syndrome (mongolism). *Clin. Chim. Acta* 25: 199, 1969.

PFLÜGER, E., Versuche der Befruchtung Überreifer Eier. *Arch. ges. Physiol.* 26: 76, 1882.

PICKERING, D. E. and D. A. FISHER, Therapeutic concepts relating to hypothyroidism in childhood. *J. chron. Dis.* 7: 242, 1958.

POLAND, B. J., Study of developmental anomalies in the spontaneously aborted fetus. *Amer. J. Obstet. Gynec.* 100: 501, 1968.

PRIEST, J. H., Parental dermatoglyphs in age-independent mongolism. *J. med. Genet.* 6: 304, 1969.

PRINDLE, R. A., TH. H. INGALLS and S. B. KIRKWOOD, Maternal hydramnios and congenital anomalies of the central nervous system. *N. Engl. J. Med.* 252: 555, 1955.

RECORD, R. G. and T. McKEOWN, Congenital malformations of the central nervous system. I. *Brit. J. soc. Med.* 3: 183, 1949.

RECORD, R. G. and T. McKEOWN, Congenital malformations of the central nervous system. II. *Ann. Eugen.* 15: 285, 1950.

RECORD, R. G. and A. SMITH, Incidence, mortality and sex distribution of mongoloid defectives. *Brit. J. prev. soc. Med.* 9: 10, 1955.

RECORD, R. G. and J. H. EDWARDS, Environmental influences related to the aetiology of congenital dislocation of the hip. *Brit. J. prev. soc. Med.* 12: 8, 1958.

ROBINSON, A., W. B. GOAD, TH. T. PUCK et al., Studies on chromosomal nondisjunction in man. III. *Amer. J. hum. Genet.* 21: 466, 1969.

144

ROBINSON, M., Failing lactation. *Lancet* i: 66, 1943.

ROSEN, F. S., The lymphocyte and the thymus gland- congenital and hereditary abnormalities. *New Engl. J. Med.* 279; 643, 1968.

ROSENBERG, I. N., Menstrual instability in thyroid disease. *Clin. Obstet. Gynec.* 12: 755, 1969.

ROSNER, F., Dermatoglyphics in leukaemia. *Lancet* ii: 882, 1970.

RUNDLE, A. T., The thyroid gland as a major causative factor in growth abnormalities of mentally retarded children. *J. ment. Defic. Res.* 15: 51, 1971.

SALBER, E. J., M. FEINLEIB and B. MACMAHON, The duration of post partum amenorrhea. *Amer. J. Epidem.* 82: 347, 1965.

SANDSTRÖM, B., Diabetes mellitus och menstruation. *Nord. Med.* 81: 727, 1969.

SCHEER, W. M. VAN DER, Over mongolismus. *Ned. Maandschr. Verlosk. Vrouwenz. en Kindergeneesk.* 8: 217, 1919.

SCHEER, W. M. VAN DER, *Beitrage zur Kenntnis der mongoloiden Missbildung.* Verlag S. Karger, Berlin, 1927.

SHAPIRO, S., L. J. ROSS and H. S. LEVINE, Relationship of selected prenatal factors to pregnancy outcome and congenital anomalies. *Amer. J. publ. Hlth* 55: 268, 1965.

SIGLER, A. T., B. H. COHEN, A. M. LILIENFELD et al., Reproductive and marital experience of parents of children with Down's syndrome (mongolism). *J. Pediat.* 70: 608, 1967.

SMILKSTEIN, G., A ten year study of anencephaly. *Calif. Med.* 96: 350, 1962.

SMITH, A. and T. MCKEOWN, Pre-natal growth of mongoloid defectives. *Arch. Dis. Childh.* 30: 257, 1955.

SMITH, A. and R. G. RECORD, Maternal age and birth rank in the aetiology of mongolism. *Brit. J. prev. soc. Med.* 9: 51, 1955, Ibidem 9: 89, 1955.

SMITH, D. W. and E. BOSTIAN, The frequency of associated congenital anomalies in children with idiopathic mental retardation. *J. Pediat.* 65: 189, 1964.

SMITH, D. W. and J. M. AASE, Polygenic inheritance of certain common malformations. *J. Pediat.* 76: 653, 1970.

SMITHELLS, R. W. and E. R. CHINN, Spina bifida in Liverpool. *Develop. Med. Child. Neurol.* 7: 258, 1965.

SOUTHAM, A. L., Disorders of menstruation. *Clin. Obstet. Gynec.* 9: 779, 1966.

STARK, C. R. and C. RUDZKI, Infectious hepatitis and Down's syndrome. *Lancet* ii: 572, 1970.

STEWART, A. L., A. J. KEAY and P. G. SMITH, Congenital malformations: a detailed study of 2.500 live born infants. *Ann. hum. Genet.* 32: 353, 1969.

STILL, G. G., Place-in-family as a factor in disease. *Lancet* ii: 853, 1927.

STOCKARD, CH. R., Developmental rate and structural expression. *Amer. J. Anat.* 28: 115, 1920–1921.

STOLLER, A. and R. D. COLLMANN, Patterns of occurrence of birth in Victoria, Australia, producing Down's syndrome (mongolism) and congenital anomalies of the central nervous system. *Med. J. Aust.* 1: 1, 1965.

STOLLER, A. and R. D. COLLMANN, Viral hepatitis and Down's syndrome. *Lancet* ii: 859, 1966.

STORRS, E. E. and R. J. WILLIAMS, A study of monozygous quadruplet armadillos in relation to mammalian inheritance. *Proc. nat. Acad. Sci.* 60: 910, 1968.

STOTT, D. H., Mongolism related to emotional shock in early pregnancy. *Vita hum.* 4: 57, 1961.

STREAN, L. P. and L. A. PEER, Stress as an etiologic factor in the development of cleft palate. *Plast. Reconstruct. Surg.* 18: 1, 1956.

STREAN, L. P., Über die Beziehungen von pränatalen Faktoren zu angeborenen Missbildungen. *Arzt. Wschr.* 13: 110, 1958.

TIMONEN, S., O. LOKKI, K. WICHMANN et al., Seasonal changes in obstetrical phenomena. *Acta obstet. gynec. scand.* 44: 507, 1965.

TIMONEN, S. and E. CARPEN, Multiple pregnancy and photoperiodicity. *Ann. Chir. et Gynec. Fenn.* 57: 135, 1968.

TOEWS, H. A. and H. W. JONES, Cyclopia in association with D trisomy and gonadal agenesis. *Amer. J. Obstet. Gynec.* 102: 53, 1968.

TOLAROVA, M., Isolated cleft palate: a genealogic study using codified genealogic questionnaire. *Cleft Palate J.* 7: 476, 1969.

TOLAROVA, M., Genealogical analysis of isolated cleft palate. *Acta Chir. plast.* 11: 801, 1969.

Tonomura, A., H. Oishi, E. Matsunaga et al., Down's syndrome: a cytogenetic and statistical survey of 127 Japanese patients. *Jap. J. hum. Genet.* 11: 1, 1966.

Turnbull, E. P. N. and J. Walker, The outcome of pregnancy, complicated by threatened abortion. *J. Obstet. Gynaec. Brit. Emp.* 63: 553, 1956.

Turpin, R. and J. Lejeune, Etude dermatoglyphique des paumes des mongoliens et de leurs parents et germains. *Sem. Hôp. Paris* 29: 3955, 1953.

Vaitukaitis, J. L. and J. C. Melby, Menstrual disorders associated with adrenal dysfunction. *Clin. Obstet. Gynec.* 12: 755, 1969.

Vanhaelst, L., F. Hayez, M. Bonnyns et al., Pathologie thyroïdienne et troubles chromosomiques. *Ann. Endocr. (Paris)* 30: 659, 1969.

Vogel, M., Lymphoreticuläre Dysgenesie bei Turner Syndrome. *Verh. dtsch. Ges. Path.* 52: 455, 1968.

Waardenburg, P. J., *Das menschliche Auge und seine Erbanlagen.* M. Nijhoff, Den Haag 1932, p 44–48.

Warkany, J. and J. L. Selkirk, Discordant monozygotic twins: hypothyroidism. *Amer. J. Dis. Child.* 89: 144, 1955.

Watts, G. F., A. W. Diddle, W. H. Gardner et al., Pregnancy following withdrawal from oral contraceptive measures. *Amer. J. Obstet. Gynec.* 90: 401, 1964.

Wertelecki, W., J. F. Fraumeni and J. J. Mulvihill, Nongonadal neoplasia in Turner's syndrome. *Cancer* 26: 485, 1970.

Wiener, G., The relationship of birth weight and length of gestation to intellectual development at ages 8 to 10 years. *J. Pediat.* 76: 694, 1970.

Wilkerson, L., J. F. Donnelly and J. A. Abernathy, Perinatal mortality and premature birth among pregnancies complicated by threatened abortion. *Amer. J. Obst. Gynec.* 96: 64, 1966.

Williams, E. D., E. Engel and A. P. Forbes, Thyroiditis and gonadal dysgenesis. *New Engl. J. Med.* 270: 805, 1964.

Witschi, E., Overripeness of the egg as a cause of twinning and teratogenesis. A review. *Cancer Res.* 12: 763, 1952.

Wolff, E. de, K. Schärer and J. Lejeune, Contribution à l'étude des jumeaux mongoliens. *Helv. Paediat. Acta* 17: 301, 1962.

Woolf, C., J. Koehn and S. Coleman, Congenital hip disease in Utah. The influence of genetic and non-genetic factors. *Amer. J. Hum. Gen.* 20: 430, 1968.

Wright, S. W., R. W. Day, H. D. Mosier et al., Klinefelter's syndrome, Down's syndrome and twinning in the same sibship. *J. Pediat.* 62: 217, 1963.

Wyshak, G., Intervals between births in families containing one set of twins. *J. biosoc. Sci.* 1: 337, 1969.

Yen, S. and B. MacMahon, Genetics of anencephaly and spina bifida? *Lancet* ii: 623, 1968.

Yerushalmy, J., J. M. Bierman, D. H. Kemp et al., Longitudinal studies of pregnancy on the island of Kauai, Territory of Hawaii. *Amer. J. Obstet. Gynec.* 71: 80, 1956.

Zajaczkowska, K., Palmar dermatoglyphics in patients with Down's syndrome and in their parents. *Pol. Med. J.* 8: 1477, 1969.

Zondek, L. H. and Th. Zondek, Observations on the testis in anencephaly with special reference to the Leydig cells. *Biol. Neonat.* 8: 329, 1965.

Curriculum Vitae

The author was born at Bruges (Belgium) on February 21st, 1933. He studied at the University of Ghent and took his degree of doctor in Medicine, Surgery and Obstetrics on July 15th 1958. During his training at the paediatric clinic of Ghent University under Professor Dr. C. Hooft, he qualified himself in clinical genetics. On July 11th, 1963, he was registered as a paediatrician. From July 1st, 1964, he has been a member of the staff of Huize 'Maria Roepaan' at Ottersum (The Netherlands) under G. van der Most, superintendent. This institute is a centre for observation and treatment of the mentally retarded. His appointment as medical director followed on October 1st, 1970.